EVIDENCE for Innovation

TRANSFORMING CHILDREN'S HEALTH THROUGH THE PHYSICAL ENVIRONMENT

A publication of the
National Association of Children's Hospitals
and Related Institutions
in collaboration with
The Center for Health Design

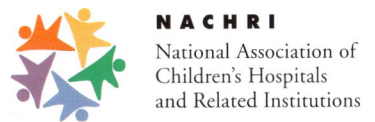
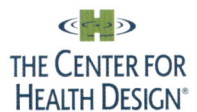

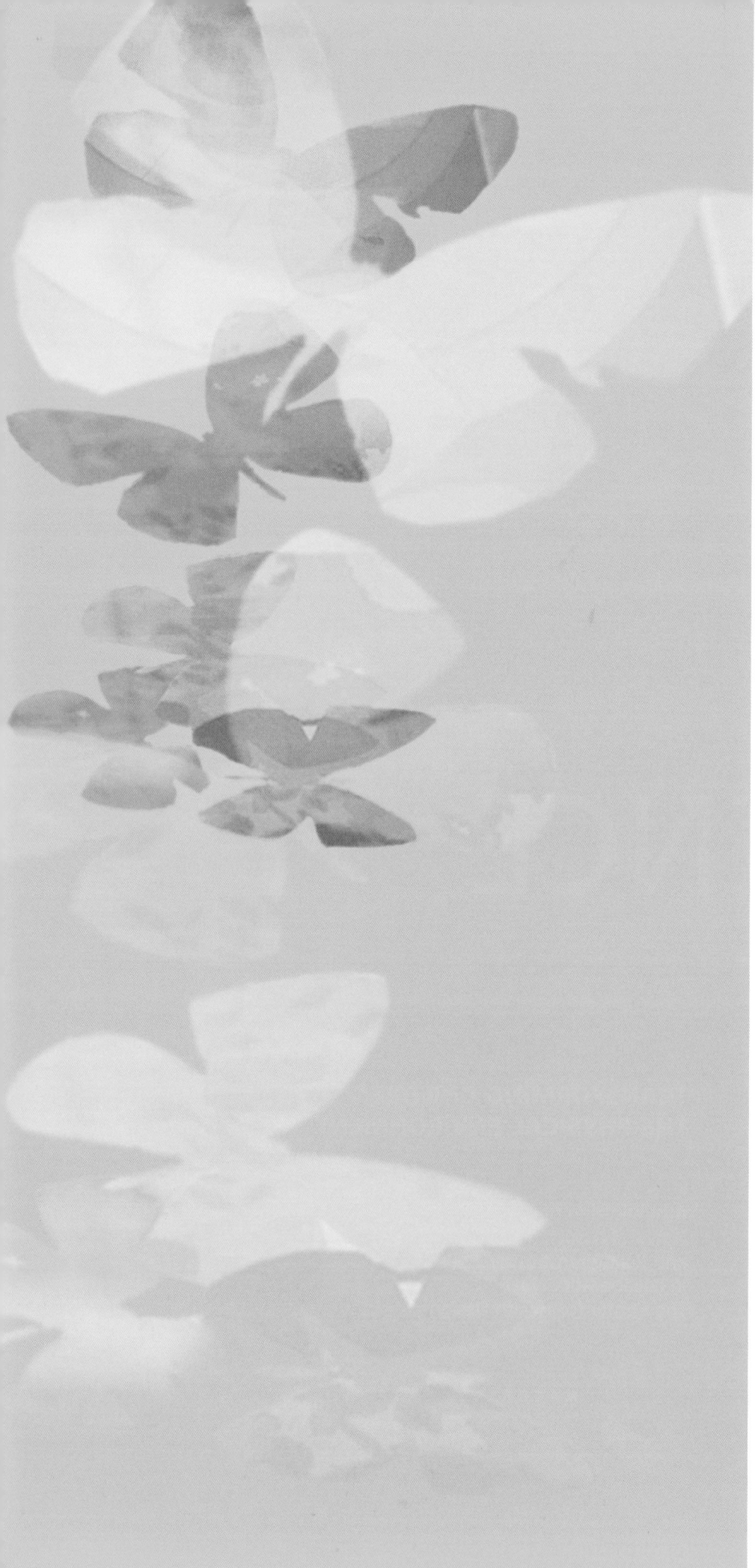

Copyright © 2008 by the National Association of Children's Hospitals and Related Institutions. All rights reserved. This publication or parts thereof may not be reproduced, distributed or transmitted in any form without the prior written permission of the publisher.

National Association of
Children's Hospitals
and Related Institutions
401 Wythe Street
Alexandria, VA 22314
703/684-1355
www.childrenshospitals.net

First Edition: June 2008
Designed by Laurie Dewhirst Young
Printed in the United States of America

ISBN-13: 978-0-9816351-0-1
ISBN-10: 0-9816351-0-5

Cover design used with permission. Rendering of a children's hospital lobby from a design competition. Courtesy of Anshen+Allen.

EVIDENCE for Innovation

| TRANSFORMING CHILDREN'S HEALTH THROUGH THE PHYSICAL ENVIRONMENT

CONTENTS

1 | INTRODUCTION
NACHRI i
Lawrence A. McAndrews, President and Chief Executive Officer, NACHRI

The Center for Health Design ii
Debra J. Levin, President and Chief Executive Officer, The Center for Health Design

Project Team iii
Blair Sadler, Project Leader, former President and Chief Executive Officer, Rady Children's Hospital, San Diego, and Senior Fellow, Institute for Healthcare Improvement

2 | EXECUTIVE SUMMARY, RECOMMENDATIONS AND CONCLUSION 1
*Blair Sadler, Project Leader, former President and Chief Executive Officer, Rady Children's Hospital, San Diego, and Senior Fellow, Institute for Healthcare Improvement
and Anjali Joseph, Ph.D., Director of Research, The Center for Health Design*

Introduction 1
Summary of Published Literature 2
Recommended Evidence-based Design Innovations 5
The Business Case Summary...12
How to Use Evidence-based Design: A Toolkit for Action..14
Conclusion 16

**3 | TRANSFORMING CARE IN CHILDREN'S HOSPITALS THROUGH
ENVIRONMENTAL DESIGN: LITERATURE REVIEW** 18
Anjali Joseph, Ph.D., Director of Research, Amy Keller, M. Arch, Research
Associate, and Katie Kronick, Project Manager, The Center for Health Design

    Study Methodology 20
    Children in Health Care Environments 21
    Advancing Patient Centered and Family Centered Care through Design 22
    Promoting Safety through Design 35
    Increase Staff Effectiveness in Providing Care through Design................................41
    Conclusions and Future Research Directions 45
    Appendix 47

4 | THE BUSINESS CASE FOR BUILDING BETTER PEDIATRIC FACILITIES..96
Blair L. Sadler, J.D., Jennifer R. DuBose, MS, LEED AP, Research Associate II,
Georgia Institute of Technology, and Craig Zimring, Ph.D., Professor of Architecture and
Psychology, Georgia Institute of Technology

    Overview 97
    Connecting Safety and Quality Improvement to the Physical Environment 98
    An Approaching Financial Tsunami – Pay for Performance...99
    Coming Soon: Hospitals Will No Longer Charge for Their Errors 100
    Patient Satisfaction and Transparency: HCAHPS Changes the Rules 101
    Balancing One-time Capital Costs and Ongoing Operating Savings.........................101
    The Cost Implications of Evidence-based Design Innovations 102
    Going Green: Another Dimension of the Business Case...105
    A Challenge: Converting "Light Green" to "Dark Green" Dollars 106
    Making It Happen: Ask Question #6 107
    From Ideas to Action: Ten Steps to Create Your Business Case............................108
    A Framework for Evaluating Evidence-based Design Features 109
    Appendix: Four Case Studies 112

REFERENCES 116

ADVISORY COMMITTEE 134

ABOUT NACHRI AND THE CENTER FOR HEALTH DESIGN.......................................135

1 | INTRODUCTION
NACHRI

The genesis of this publication grew from a conversation that I had with Blair Sadler, former president and chief executive officer of Rady Children's Hospital, San Diego, and senior fellow at the Institute for Healthcare Improvement.

We were discussing a literature review linking the physical design of adult health care facilities with patient and staff outcomes when the concept of a similar report for pediatric facilities emerged. The link between the design of the physical environment and quality improvement has been well documented in adult care, but there had been no comprehensive look at the building environments in pediatric facilities, in particular children's hospitals.

Until now.

In 2007, NACHRI partnered with The Center for Health Design to begin the research process for this landmark report. Based on a scientific review of 320 articles in the literature, *Evidence for Innovation* provides an in-depth look at the outcomes of applying evidence-based design in pediatric settings and makes strong recommendations that will help children's hospitals, large and small, improve the quality of the care that they provide.

In addition, this publication presents the business case for evidence-based design and demonstrates that children's hospitals cannot afford to sit on the sidelines of this approach given the compelling financial and health care implications for children, especially not when family centered care can be strengthened, pediatric outcomes improved, infection rates decreased, efficiency enhanced and staff morale boosted.

Now is the time for children's hospitals to evaluate where they are on the path to using every credible resource available to innovate and transform children's health care for the better. This publication is one such resource. NACHRI commends the children's hospitals that have already taken up the charge to improve care through evidence-based design and challenges those hospitals not yet engaged to contribute to advancing the science.

Lawrence A. McAndrews, FACHE
President and Chief Executive Officer
National Association of
Children's Hospitals
and Related Institutions

INTRODUCTION
THE CENTER FOR HEALTH DESIGN

Recent years have seen a growing desire for empirical evidence to validate our intuition that the physical environment can impact outcomes in health care settings. As the industry advances, evidence mounts that thoughtful facility design can help bring patients, staff and families into the center of the health care experience, increases safety, encourages family participation, supports an already overburdened staff and advances the overall quality of care provided.

These types of buildings are exactly what we should aspire to build for pediatric settings because design can truly support children in a unique way. Design as a fundamental element can bring about change in the way health care is provided and experienced by all in children's health care settings.

Children's hospitals have a level of design quality and sophistication not seen in other areas of health care. As more pediatric facilities are built, it is critical that we continue to use the best and most current information available to guide the process.

Evidence for Innovation is the comprehensive tool for children's hospital administrators, architects and designers. This publication provides cutting edge research information on how building design can impact outcomes in pediatric settings; and it presents evidence-based recommendations and a roadmap for implementing these changes. In addition, it dispenses valuable information for all facilities seeking change – whether alterations to a pre-existing structure, new construction or major renovation is planned. The clearly argued business case strongly supports financial justification for implementing evidence-based design in pediatric facilities.

The Center for Health Design is proud to have partnered with the National Association of Children's Hospitals and Related Institutions on this project. Supporting others to make design decisions influenced by research has always been the basis of our work. It is our hope that this publication becomes another valuable resource for doing just that.

Debra J. Levin
President and Chief Executive Officer
The Center for Health Design

INTRODUCTION
PROJECT TEAM

When Larry McAndrews first suggested that the National Association of Children's Hospitals and Related Institutions embark on this project in partnership with The Center for Health Design, I thought the timing could not be better. Many pediatric facilities are currently undertaking construction and renovation projects. The demands on all hospitals to provide optimally healing environments have never been greater. The field of evidence-based design (like evidence-based medicine) is exploding with new research and ideas. The green revolution has arrived, and a strong business case for utilizing evidence-based design now exists.

We have been greatly assisted in building this academic exploration of evidence-base design by a dedicated and diverse multidisciplinary advisory committee. Committee members have contributed numerous ideas and comments to truly energize and enhance this work. A dedicated working group from NACHRI and The Center for Health Design was essential to organizing and completing the effort. Members of the advisory committee and working group are listed at the end of the publication.

It is an exciting time to build new facilities and improve our existing ones. Just imagine: a future where all children, their families and hospital staffs work in quiet, calming, uncluttered, easy-to-find, harm-free environments that are truly patient centered (private whenever appropriate) and absolutely minimize patient transfers from unit to unit or floor to floor. Imagine that through inexpensive innovations in music and art, each child and family can control some of their environment.

I believe we all share the vision that a child who is in our care for an hour, a day, a week or a year deserves to be treated in an optimal healing environment.

I hope that this book helps you in your journey of evidence-based design on behalf of the children we serve.

Blair L. Sadler, J.D.
Project Leader
Past President and Chief Executive Officer
Rady Children's Hospital, San Diego
Senior Fellow, Institute for Healthcare Improvement

Executive Summary

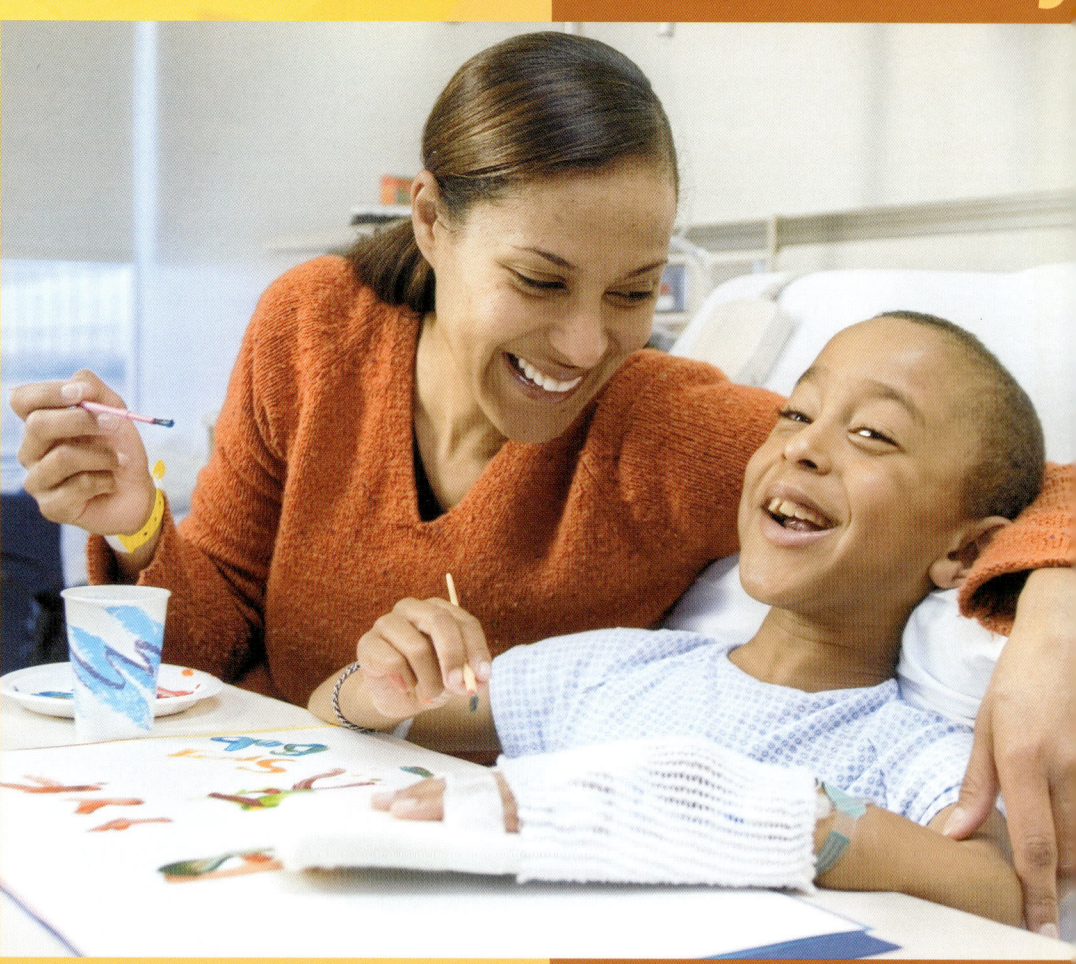

Mother and son bond on the road to recovery.
Photo by Leonard Myszynski, Solar Eye Photography
Children's Hospital of Orange County, Orange, CA

BLAIR L. SADLER, J.D.
Past President and Chief Executive Officer
Rady Children's Hospital, San Diego
Senior Fellow, Institute for Healthcare Improvement

ANJALI JOSEPH, Ph.D.
Director of Research
The Center for Health Design

Evidence-based design is defined as the deliberate attempt to base building decisions on the best available evidence with the goal of achieving the best possible outcomes for patients, families and staff while improving utilization of resources.

We are currently in the midst of an unprecedented health care building boom with $100 billion in inflation-adjusted dollars spent on new hospital construction in the past five years (K. Henriksen, S. Isaacson, B. Sadler, & C. Zimring, 2007). Children's hospitals are part of this trend to upgrade, expand or replace existing facilities. The key drivers for this include: age of existing facilities (built in the 1950s-1960s) that no longer support efficient and safe care delivery; advances in treating childhood diseases; rapidly emerging technologies that fundamentally change care delivery processes; and the growing importance of patient and family centered care. Most importantly, the heightened focus on improving patient and workforce safety and quality has increased the need to create optimal physical environments.

In its landmark 2001 report, *Crossing the Quality Chasm,* the Institute of Medicine identified several problems with the health care system in the United States: that it was unsafe, ineffective, inefficient, untimely, lacking patient centeredness and not equitable (Institute of Medicine, 2000, 2001). Since then, a patient safety and quality revolution has swept the country. Consumers, employers and payers are demanding that hospitals dramatically reduce system-based errors that harm, even kill thousands of patients annually (Sadler, 2006). Further, negative outcomes such as patient falls, nosocomial infections, medical errors and staff turnover significantly impact costs of providing care. Universal health care access and escalating costs have emerged as a top issue in national and local political campaigns.

A growing body of research shows that the physical design of health care settings unintentionally contributes to negative outcomes. On the other hand, thoughtful evidence-based facility design can help bring the patient, staff and families into the center of the health care experience, increase patient safety and enhance the overall quality of care provided. For example, as part of a comprehensive quality improvement program, the physical environment can help to eliminate avoidable harmful conditions such as hospital-acquired infections that cost hospitals millions of dollars. (Agency for Healthcare Research and Quality, 2007; Clancy, 2008; K. Henriksen, S. Isaacson, B. L. Sadler, & C. M. Zimring, 2007).

It has become imperative to rethink facility design as a critical element in bringing about change in the way health care is provided and experienced in children's health care settings. Evidence-based design links the design of the physical environment with an organization's patient safety and quality improvement agenda. *Evidence-based design is defined as the deliberate attempt to base building decisions on the best available evidence with the goal of achieving the best possible outcomes for patients, families and staff while improving utilization of resources.* When the significant, multiyear, reduced operating costs of harm avoided are considered, there is a powerful business case for evidence-based design. Emerging trends in reimbursement and publicly reported patient satisfaction scores will further strengthen the business case.

Evidence for Innovation brings together key elements that can help leaders of children's hospitals to take action to create safer, less stressful and more patient centered healing environments. It consists of:
- *Key evidence-based design recommendations* that hospital leaders can incorporate in new, renovated or existing facilities (full report)
- *A tool kit* that outlines the key steps to take in implementing evidence-based hospital design
- *A comprehensive literature review* of evidence of the impact of the physical environment on patient, family and staff outcomes in children's hospitals
- *A business case analysis* that enables pediatric leaders to understand the cost benefits of investing in evidence-based environmental design strategies, including a suggested framework for return on investment.

SUMMARY OF PUBLISHED LITERATURE

The literature review clearly demonstrates that the physical environment of pediatric settings impacts clinical, developmental, psychosocial and safety outcomes among patients and families. The physical environment represents a key component in providing family centered care in pediatric settings.

A scientific literature review identified the empirical evidence linking the design of the physical environment with patient, staff and family outcomes in pediatric health care settings. The literature review primarily focused on empirical studies published in scientific peer-reviewed journals. Of the 450 studies found on initial search using keywords, 320 articles met the criteria for inclusion in this study. Of these, 223 are cited in the literature review. Seventy-eight articles were analyzed in detail, and that analysis forms the core of the full report, *Evidence for Innovation*.

The review covers a range of pediatric services along the continuum of care and involving different patient populations. Of these, the greatest amount of research looking at impacts on patients, families and staff has been conducted in neonatal intensive care units (NICU). The key findings from the literature review are summarized here. For a more detailed review of the research findings and references, see the full report.

Improved clinical and physiological outcomes in the NICU

The fragile state of the patients in the NICU makes them especially vulnerable to the harmful effects of environmental factors such as loud noise, high light levels and infectious pathogens. Exposure to excessive noise in the NICU impacts short-term and long-term auditory development. Removing sources of loud noises, instituting quiet hours, educating staff and parents, putting in sound absorbing ceiling tiles and flooring and providing single patient rooms (as opposed to open wards) are all effective in reducing noise levels. Additional interventions demonstrating physiological benefits for infant development and convalescence include: placing earmuffs on the infants, covering the incubator, installing a sound absorbing panel in the incubator and putting sound absorbing foam next to the infant.

Cycled lighting (reduced light levels at night) and providing focused lighting over incubators helps to improve sleep and developmental outcomes among infants. Light is also beneficial in treating neonatal jaundice.

Many new NICU designs are moving from open wards to single family rooms with the primary purpose of providing an environment that can be customized to the developmental/health needs of the infant. Some studies suggest that families and staff are also more satisfied in these environments while others indicate that open bays may have some advantages related to ease of staff monitoring. Additional research is needed in this area.

Improved clinical outcomes

Loud noise levels are common in general pediatric settings as well, and strategies such as providing single patient rooms and closing room doors have shown to be effective in reducing noise levels. There is, however, a lack of studies examining the impacts of noise on young children, adolescents or families on pediatric units.

Studies conducted in inpatient and outpatient settings show that positive distractions such as noise reduction and choice of music using a headset can be helpful in reducing anxiety, distress and perceived pain associated with difficult procedures. Music and music therapy is also an effective intervention in reducing stress, anxiety, perceived pain and the need for conscious sedation among hospitalized and ambulatory patients. One study that examined the impact of music therapy on the need for sedation among children receiving ECGs (electrocardiograms) or CT (computed tomography) scans found 100 percent success rate in eliminating the need for sedation for pediatric patients receiving ECGs, 80.7 percent success rate for pediatric CT scan completion without sedation and a 94.1 percent success rate for all other procedures (Walworth, 2005). Savings per patient was $74.20, and total savings for 92 patients was $6,830 (Walworth, 2005).

Spending time in gardens is also effective in improving mood, reducing distress and increasing feelings of wellness among young children. Other studies show that healing among children is promoted through interior design elements such as color, furniture and carpet while use of ambient music can help patients cope with pain and aggression.

Improved psychosocial outcomes

Providing spaces for families on nursing units and in patient rooms enables parents, siblings and friends to spend time with patients and provide the social interaction and support needed during this difficult time. Well designed positive distraction tools such as Starlight Starbright programs help school-age children connect with a community of peers and provide much needed social contact and intellectual stimulation. Studies show the therapeutic benefits of providing play spaces in health care settings to support play behavior and interaction among patients with different types of physical abilities and ages.

Adolescents have different social needs from younger children. Adolescent patients require a balance between privacy and intimacy and social interaction with people. Programmed amenities (game rooms, music areas) that provide distraction and remove the feeling of being in a hospital are likely to be preferred by adolescent patients.

Increased patient safety

Patient safety outcomes such as nosocomial infections and falls are directly impacted by environmental factors. Poor air quality, inadequate supports for hand washing and materials (e.g., toys) harboring infectious pathogens have all been linked with nosocomial infections in children. Research shows that single patient rooms are more effective than open bays in reducing the spread of nosocomial infection among pediatric patients, especially among immunocompromised patients.

Environmental factors potentially contribute to falls in children although no studies have examined this in any detail. Other environmental hazards such as bedrails, wires and equipment that could lead to choking, tripping or burns among children should also be avoided. The physical environment can also compromise patient safety. For example, loud noises and inadequate meeting spaces are barriers to communication and team work. Chaotic environments, poor ergonomics and low lighting levels may compound the burden of stress in staff and result in errors. These studies have been primarily conducted in adult settings, but are applicable to pediatric settings.

Increased staff effectiveness in providing care

Satisfied and effective personnel are integral components to providing quality care in pediatric hospitals, although few studies have focused specifically on staff outcomes in children's health care environments. However, findings from studies conducted with staff in adult settings likely apply to pediatric settings. Excessive noise is a stressor for staff and leads to fatigue and burnout. In contrast, exposure to gardens is a source of satisfaction, improved mood and reduced stress. Some studies have examined the impact of unit design and interior design changes on staff satisfaction. They suggest that staff prefers and has less stress in single family rooms in the NICU. However, in some cases, staff members in NICUs have expressed concerns with single patient room designs believing that they make monitoring and effectively caring for patients more difficult. Unit renovations and physical design improvements are associated with greater staff satisfaction. Some studies conducted in adult settings suggest that unit layouts result in increased efficiency when designed to reduce walking, to increase staff access to patients, and to place equipment and supplies closer to staff. However, there is need for further research in pediatric settings.

In summary, research studies in various pediatric environments show how physical design can contribute to safety and quality. Many other studies on adult settings are also applicable to pediatrics. A strong body of information is now available to guide design decision makers in creating safe and therapeutic pediatric health care environments. Further research in pediatric settings is needed and is worthy of support to assure that our children are receiving optimal care. Based on the literature review, we recommend six key areas where further research is needed.

Key areas where future research is needed on designing for children and adolescents

- Role of design in reducing noise levels and associated negative outcomes
- Effect of natural light in reducing depression and improving outcomes
- Impact of unit design (i.e., decentralization) and patient room design on staff time at the bedside and staff efficiency
- Impact of unit design and acuity adaptable room design on patient transfers and errors
- Impact of positive distractions such as artwork and music on stress reduction and anxiety
- Cost effectiveness of various design innovations

RECOMMENDED EVIDENCE-BASED DESIGN INNOVATIONS

While the body of research on the impact of the physical environment on patient, staff and family outcomes in pediatric settings continues to grow, the stronger focus has been on NICU settings as compared to environments for pediatric and adolescent patients. Although children and adolescents often have different physical and psychosocial needs from adult patients, in many areas, research from adult settings is applicable to pediatrics. For example, a strong body of research from adult settings shows that optimal exposure to sunlight is beneficial in reducing depression and perceptions of pain among adult patients. Although similar research has not been conducted among children and adolescents, it stands to reason that sunlight should also benefit these populations.

Some new trends in the design of health care settings – pediatric and adult – are not yet fully substantiated by research, but are extremely promising. As leaders of pediatric health care organizations embark on construction, renovation or physical improvement projects, they should consider the following evidence-based design strategies organized in three categories:
- Evidence-based design strategies from pediatric settings (NICU, children and adolescents)
- Evidence-based design strategies from adult settings applicable in pediatric settings
- Promising high impact strategies not yet fully substantiated by research

The evidence-based design strategies are organized as a matrix in Table 1 on page 6. Strategies for each of the three categories are indicated in terms of:
- *Relevance to a specific population* – the population directly impacted by the evidence-based design strategy. While indirect impacts on other groups are likely, *Evidence for Innovation* focuses on the direct impacts as indicated by the research literature.
- *Relative construction costs* – the costs of incorporating this strategy relative to other strategies. A wide range of costs reflects the scale of changes and whether the strategy is to be incorporated in a new facility or in a renovation. The range describes: low = less than $100,000; moderate = $100,000 to $1 million; and high = more than $1million.
- *When to incorporate* – the types of situations (new construction, renovation or existing facility) when the evidence-based design strategy can be cost effectively incorporated into the physical environment.

Evidence-based design strategies based on research in pediatric settings

The following strategies have proven effective in pediatric-specific settings. The timing and relative cost of the intervention are included.

Construct single family rooms in the NICU
☐ New construction/renovation
☐ High cost

Studies show that single family rooms are beneficial in the NICU because they allow a greater degree of flexibility to care providers and families in customizing the environment (noise levels, lighting and temperature) needed for the care of a specific patient (Harris, Shepley, White, Kolberg, & Harrell, 2006). These single family enclosed rooms include a patient care area (with incubator), a staff area (sinks, storage) and a separate family area (usually with sleeping space, workspace). Patient and family privacy is supported by having curtains/doors at the entrance to the room and curtains between the patient area and family area. Families and staff are also more satisfied in these environments as

EXECUTIVE SUMMARY

TABLE 1

Evidence Based Design Strategies	Relevance to population						Construction cost			When to incorporate		
	General/all	NICU	PICU/pediatric	Adolescent	Staff	Families	Low	Moderate	High	New construction	Renovation	Existing
Strategies from pediatric settings												
Single family room NICU		■				■			■	■	■	
Circadian lighting in the NICU		■						■		■	■	■
Incubator noise reduction in the NICU		■					■			■	■	■
Sound absorbing ceiling tiles	■							■		■	■	■
Space for families in all patient rooms and on all units	■					■		■		■	■	
Patient and family control over privacy and environmental conditions		■	■	■		■		■		■	■	■
Calming music distractions before/during procedures		■	■	■			■			■	■	■
Positive distractions to reduce anxiety		■	■	■			■			■	■	■
Access to nature through gardens	■							■		■	■	
Age appropriate play areas			■	■				■		■	■	■
Overall ambience and attractiveness	■							■		■	■	■
Applicable strategies from adult settings												
Effective way finding systems	■							■		■	■	■
Single patient rooms for all patients	■								■	■	■	
Hand washing dispensers and sinks in every room	■				■			■		■	■	■
Access to natural light	■							■		■	■	
Ceiling lifts					■			■		■	■	■
Noise audits	■						■			■	■	■
Visual access and accessibility to patient	■				■			■		■	■	
Positive distractions	■						■			■	■	■
HEPA filtration for immune-compromised patients		■	■					■		■	■	■
Promising high impact strategies not fully substantiated by research												
Acuity adaptable patient rooms	■								■	■	■	
Increased standardization through same-handed patient rooms	■							■		■	■	
Increased standardization through consistent room and unit layout	■							■		■	■	

compared to open bay NICUs. Single family rooms are best incorporated into the facility during unit renovations or new construction because of the extensive modifications required.

Incorporate circadian lighting in the NICU
☐ Any time
☐ Low cost

Research shows that when light levels are changed over the course of the day to mimic night and day cycles, infants show improved developmental outcomes such as improved sleep and weight gain. This low cost strategy can be incorporated any time. Single family rooms offer greater flexibility in terms of controlling light levels in the NICU to accommodate differing lighting needs of patients, staff and families.

Incorporate incubator noise reduction in the NICU
☐ Any time
☐ Low cost

Altering noise levels within an infant's incubator can be an efficient low cost way to alter the noise environment and may not require facility renovations. Placing earmuffs on the infants, covering the incubator, installing a sound absorbing panel in the incubator and putting sound absorbing foam next to the infant all have demonstrated physiological benefits for infant development and convalescence.

Install sound-absorbing ceiling tiles
☐ Any time
☐ Low cost

This relatively low cost strategy has proven effective in improving the acoustical environment by reducing noise levels and reverberation times. While only a few studies have been conducted in pediatric settings, the cost effectiveness of this strategy in reducing noise levels makes it a good solution in many health care settings. Further, this strategy can be incorporated in any situation. An acoustical consultant can provide input on placement and selection of tiles to achieve maximum effectiveness.

Provide space for families
☐ New construction/renovation
☐ Moderate/high cost

To help children cope with their hospital experiences, family members can provide distractions, emotional and verbal expression, independent activities, familiarity and knowledge. Providing ample family space in each patient room to encourage parents and siblings to remain with the child can result in ongoing support. Single family rooms with space for families are the most supportive of family presence. It is easier to incorporate such family spaces when units are being constructed or renovated. However, even in existing facilities, spaces can sometimes be created for family use.

Provide patient and family control over privacy
☐ Any time
☐ Moderate cost

Multiple studies demonstrate patients' needs for privacy as well as the ability to control their environments. While single patient rooms provide the greatest opportunity for individualization and privacy, small scale interventions such as individual storage space and furniture partitions between beds can help to promote privacy in multi-occupancy conditions. Adolescents particularly indicate a strong preference for privacy and the ability to control with whom they interact and when.

Provide calming music distractions
☐ Any time
☐ Low cost

Music therapy and ambient music are effective and efficient non-pharmacological strategies in reducing anxiety, perception of pain and medication use among pediatric patients undergoing painful procedures. They can be introduced at any time.

Provide positive distractions to reduce anxiety
☐ Any time
☐ Low cost

Virtual reality games and programs have been used during painful procedures to decrease pain perception. Such interventions have been shown to be effective in reducing pain and anxiety and symptom distress. Other programs such as the computerized network Starbright World were created to link seriously ill children into an interactive online virtual community that enables them to play games, talk about their illness or learn about their condition with other chronically ill children. Since the inception of Starbright World, several research studies have shown improved outcomes: reduction in pain and distress, reduction in the fear and isolation of a prolonged illness, greater willingness to return for treatment, increased sense of peer support, increased knowledge and sense of responsibility for managing disease, distraction from the challenges that accompany their illnesses and increased ability to cope with their diseases.

Provide access to nature through gardens
☐ New construction/renovation
☐ Moderate cost

Exposure to nature in different forms (viewing nature, gardens, being in nature) have all shown a calming and restorative effect on pediatric patients as well as staff and families. Exposure to gardens has potentially beneficial effects on emotional states, feelings of anxiety, sadness, anger, worry and pain. Gardens are easier to incorporate in new construction although they could be incorporated into existing facilities if space permits. This is a moderate cost intervention.

Provide age appropriate play areas
☐ Any time
☐ Low to moderate cost

Play, used as a therapeutic tool, reduces tension, anxiety, anger, frustration and conflict among pediatric patients and provides a means for children to "play out" frightening, stressful or frustrating experiences. Age appropriate play areas are recommended on all children's units. Needs and preferences of children of different age groups as well as therapy goals should be considered when designing these spaces.

Enhance overall ambience and attractiveness
☐ Any time
☐ Low to moderate cost

Several studies show that patients, staff and families are more satisfied with the overall care in pleasant, clean and attractive settings. Even small design modification and unit renovations have been associated with increased satisfaction among staff. The cost of making a setting more attractive will vary depending on the scale of the modifications. Adding plants, paint or artwork to an existing unit would be low cost while interior design modification for the entire facility would be moderate to high cost.

Evidence-based design strategies applicable from research in adult settings

Incorporate effective way finding systems
☐ Any time
☐ Moderate cost

Poor way finding systems cause stress and disorientation for patients, families and visitors. Further, hospitals incur significant costs associated with having staff provide directions to ameliorate way finding problems. A good way finding system includes four main components working at different levels:
- administrative and procedural levels — mail-out maps, pre-visit hospital information
- external building cues — signage and location of parking, local you-are-here maps
- signage at key decision points — directories, nomenclature
- global structure — simple and accessible building layout

While overall building layout changes are feasible only in new construction projects, other components are low cost modifications, which can be incorporated in existing settings.

Provide single patient rooms for all patients
☐ New construction/renovation
☐ High cost

Research reveals that adult patients recover faster in private rooms, and infection rates are lower due to lack of exposure to airborne pathogens originating from a roommate. Medication errors are reduced due to less confusion about which patient, and privacy issues are reduced when confidential patient information is not shared in close proximity to others. Additional documented benefits of all private patient rooms include: far less noise, better communication from staff to patients and from patients to staff, superior accommodations for family, and consistently higher satisfaction with overall quality of care. There is also strong indication that single patient rooms result in better outcomes among NICU and PICU patients. Studies among adolescents indicate a preference for single rooms. Based on this converging body of evidence, we recommend single patient rooms for all patients in pediatric settings. This intervention is best considered in new construction.

Provide hand washing dispensers and sinks
☐ Any time
☐ Low cost

Several studies show that alcohol-based hand rubs in addition to sinks with soap and water in patient rooms increase the quality and frequency of hand washing. Further, alcohol-based hand-rub dispensers at the bedside are associated with increased hand washing compliance. This low cost intervention should be incorporated into any existing facility.

Optimize access to natural light
☐ New construction
☐ Moderate cost

Studies of hospitalized adults show that exposure to light helps to reduce depression, intake of pain medication and length of stay. Exposure to light might have similar benefits for children and adolescents. New construction provides the best opportunity to bring natural light indoors. This is more difficult to achieve in existing facilities.

Install ceiling lifts
☐ Any time
☐ Moderate cost

Ceiling lifts have been very effective in reducing back injuries among staff in adult settings. With growing obesity among children, it is likely that ceiling lifts will effectively reduce lifting injuries to staff in some pediatric settings as well.

Develop a noise reduction plan
☐ Any time
☐ Low cost

Noise audits can help a health care facility assess noise levels as well as sources of noise in and around the facility. An effective noise audit will provide valuable information that can lead to a comprehensive noise reduction plan including low cost solutions to specific noise problems (remove ice maker from the unit, train staff to reduce conversation levels, eliminate overhead pages, install ceiling tiles).

Promote visual access and accessibility
☐ New construction
☐ High cost

Bringing staff and supplies closer to patients is likely to reduce staff time spent walking and increase time spent in direct patient care activities. Studies on the impact of the unit layout on the amount of time spent walking show that time saved walking translates to more time spent on patient care activities and interaction with family members. New designs are incorporating decentralized nurses stations and alcoves outside patient rooms so staff is distributed around the unit (as opposed to being in a single central location) closer to the patients. Consider work flows in relation to location of key spaces (patient room, nurse work space, location of equipment and supplies) with the goal of minimizing walking distances and number of trips; consider locating frequently used supplies in patient rooms to minimize walking trips for staff.

Provide positive distractions
☐ Any time
☐ Low cost

Viewing artwork depicting images of nature has been linked to stress reduction for diverse groups of people. Studies conducted among adult patients show that viewing nature images (water, trees, large outdoor space) results in reduced anxiety and pain. A preliminary study conducted with children in a pediatric emergency department suggests that interactive art cart programs helped substantially in reducing their stress and anxiety. This low cost intervention can be incorporated into any type of pediatric facility.

Install HEPA filtration
☐ New construction/renovation
☐ Moderate cost

Several studies show that high-efficiency particulate air (HEPA) filters, in particular, are highly effective in filtering out harmful pathogens and are very helpful in reducing nosocomial infections, particularly among immunocompromised patients. Some special precautions to prevent infection during periods of construction and renovation include using portable HEPA filters and installing barriers between patient care and construction areas.

Promising high impact strategies not fully substantiated by research

Make single patient rooms acuity adaptable
☐ New construction/renovation
☐ Low cost

Acuity adaptable rooms do not cost significantly more than regular single patient rooms. Additional costs include providing monitoring and oxygen so that care can be provided in the same room for patients with differing levels of acuity and thus eliminate the need for transfers. The path breaking study conducted by Hendrich and colleagues on the impact of acuity adaptable rooms on patient transfers in adult ICU settings provides strong justification for adopting acuity adaptable room and care models as a way to reduce patient transfers in the hospital (Hendrich, Fay, & Sorrells, 2004; Hendrich & Lee, 2005). Significant improvement in many key areas was reported as a result of the acuity adaptable model: patient transfers decreased by 90 percent; medication errors decreased by 70 percent; and number of falls was drastically reduced. However, this study has not been replicated in other settings – adult or pediatric. There is reason to believe this concept would be equally effective in reducing unnecessary transfers in pediatric settings, but research is needed to understand more about how this approach should be adapted to pediatrics.

Increase standardization using same-handed rooms
☐ New construction
☐ Moderate cost

Many new designs in adult hospitals are incorporating same-handed patient rooms with all rooms identical in configuration and orientation. That is, the patient is always on the same side in all patient rooms and gases and equipment are always located in the same position in every room. The premise for this design innovation is based on human factors research from other industries showing that increased standardization results in fewer mistakes because it reduces the cognitive burden on the decision maker. However, this innovation has a higher initial capital cost, and its effectiveness remains to be proven.

Increase standardization using consistent layout
☐ New construction
☐ Moderate cost

Hospitals are aiming toward greater standardization in all aspects of their designs and operations. This means standard location, design and use for specific building components throughout the organization. For example, nurses might be able to locate certain types of supplies at specific locations consistently throughout the facility. The goal is to minimize variability, which requires staff to spend precious time and effort reorienting to new physical situations to address problems at hand. The impact of a higher degree of standardization on staff efficiency and medical errors remains to be substantiated by research.

Priority Design Recommendations

The following design recommendations have been developed based on their impact and the strength of the evidence available (Table 2). Some recommendations can be incorporated into any pediatric facility at low cost without significant modification (left column). All facilities could implement them at any time. Other strategies require higher investment and significant physical modifications and are best incorporated as part of a major renovation or new construction (right column). Leaders of pediatric facilities should seriously consider these key design strategies as integral to quality improvement projects.

TABLE 2

Priority Design Recommendations

Any time	During renovation or new construction
• Install hand washing dispensers at each bedside and in all high patient volume areas	• Build single family patient rooms
• Install incubator noise reduction measures in the NICU	• Provide adequate space for families to stay overnight in patient rooms
• Install circadian (cycled) lighting in the NICU	• Build accessible indoor or outdoor gardens
• Install high performance sound absorbing ceiling tiles	• Design age appropriate and attractive play areas and amenities
• Conduct a noise audit and develop a noise reduction plan	• Increase visual access and accessibility to patients
• Use music as a positive distraction during procedures	• Optimize natural light in staff and patient areas
• Use virtual reality images and artwork to provide positive distractions	• Install HEPA filters in all areas housing immunocompromised patients
• Incorporate age appropriate play areas	• Install effective way finding systems
• Improve way finding through enhanced signage	• Install ceiling lifts to reduce workforce injuries
• Where structurally feasible, install HEPA filters in areas housing immunocompromised patients	• Explore the feasibility of acuity adaptable rooms to reduce transfers*

*Limited evidence but potentially high impact

THE BUSINESS CASE SUMMARY
Revenue and Cost Impacts

When considering reduced operating costs and revenue enhancements, a powerful business case supports making intelligent evidence-based design decisions described in *Evidence for Innovation*. To fully appreciate this, it is important to consider the implications of several major forces beginning to change reimbursement formulas and require public reporting of quality/safety outcomes as well as comparable patient satisfaction scores.

Pay for performance

In the past few years, a fundamentally new concept has begun to emerge in the reimbursement to hospitals and physicians. It is called value-based purchasing or pay for performance, and it promises to have an important influence on the business case for quality improvement, including the physical environment where people work and care is received. While much of the emphasis so far has been on Medicare patients (driven by Centers for Medicare & Medicaid Services [CMS]), it seems safe to assume that Medicaid, the number one volume payer of children's hospitals, and commercial payers will follow in this direction. Indeed, some have already begun.

National Quality Forum "never events"

The National Quality Forum (NQF) has identified 27 "never events" that are largely preventable and should simply never occur in hospitals (National Quality Forum, 2006-07). CMS has identified specific harms, including infections and falls that should not be reimbursed. While the details are just emerging, it seems reasonable to assume that, within three to five years, virtually no payers will reimburse hospitals and physicians for serious harm caused by the care provider. Consumers will have easier access to clear, comparable outcomes data and will begin to make choices about where to take their children for care based on this information. Increasingly, consumers will be channeled to payer-preferred networks based on quality measures. Poorly performing hospitals could risk losing significant market share.

Hospitals will no longer charge for errors

In this new era of transparency and public reporting, hospitals in some states have voluntarily decided not to charge payers and patients for errors caused by the care provider. In addition, the connection between hospital errors and the incidence of litigation has been effectively described (Gosfield & Reinertsen, 2005).

Several state hospital associations have adopted a "no charge" policy for hospital-caused errors and this may soon become standard practice. We are entering a new era in which patients and payers will no longer tolerate being charged for poor outcomes.

Patient satisfaction and transparency

Another emerging trend is the mandated reporting of patient experiences in hospitals. With support from CMS and the Agency for Healthcare Research and Quality, a survey, Hospital Consumer Assessment of Healthcare Providers and Systems (HCAHPS) was developed to:
- *produce comparable data* from the patient's perspective on topics important to consumers
- *create incentives* through public reporting for hospitals to improve care
- *increase public accountability* through increased transparency of quality of care

The survey is composed of 27 items, 18 of which encompass critical aspects of the hospital experience including cleanliness and quietness of the hospital environment as well as overall rating of the hospital.

While there are no data yet to report the impact of this new trend, it seems reasonable to predict that those hospitals with more comfortable, safe and patient centered physical environments will be rated higher by patients in the HCAHPS survey. This could have significant influence on patient choice of hospitals with a resulting effect on a hospital's market share and its financial bottom line. While HCAHPS is focused today on Medicare beneficiaries, it also seems reasonable to assume that Medicaid and commercial payers will again follow and that this type of public reporting requirement will apply to children's hospitals.

These four trends combine to send a clear signal that children's hospitals could experience significant negative revenue consequences secondary to providing less than optimal environments that contribute to unacceptable clinical outcomes, lower patient satisfaction scores and reduced market share.

Balancing one-time capital costs and ongoing operating savings

Central to the business case is the need to balance one time construction costs against ongoing operating savings and revenue enhancements. The first attempt to analyze this balance was published in 2004 by a multidisciplinary team, which analyzed published research on the actual experience of health care organizations using evidence-based design in portions of construction projects including Pebble Projects supported by The Center for Health Design. The team designed the hypothetical Fable Hospital. When the team analyzed the operating cost savings resulting from reducing infections, eliminating unnecessary patient transfers, minimizing patient falls, lowering drug costs, lessening employee turnover rates, as well as improving market share and philanthropy, it concluded that, with effective management and monitoring, the financial operating benefits would continue for several years, making the additional innovations a sound long-term investment. In short, there was a compelling business case for building better, safer hospitals. While Fable Hospital was largely based on adult patients and research involving adults, a significant majority of components also apply to pediatric patients and their hospital environments.

Going green

In addition to evidence-based design features that attend to patient and staff safety, a number of emerging sustainable or "green" building features and strategies can improve the health care environment with little or no capital cost and should be considered for inclusion in new projects.

From "light green" to "dark green"

The movement of theoretical savings (light green dollars) to actual savings as reflected in hospital financial statements (dark green dollars) is a key success factor to accomplish the business case objectives. Documenting actual cost savings in financial forecasts can be invaluable in convincing boards of trustees that evidence-based design investments are cost effective.

A suggested framework for hospitals to calculate the return on investment of a specific evidence-based innovation is included in the full report, *Evidence for Innovation*. Each organization will need to incorporate the latest relevant evidence and use best judgment about cost and revenue impacts of the innovation being considered.

HOW TO USE EVIDENCE-BASED DESIGN
A Toolkit for Action

When planning to build a new hospital or to renovate an existing facility, children's hospital leaders should address a key question: How will the proposed project incorporate all relevant and proven evidence-based design innovations in order to optimize patient safety, quality and satisfaction as well as workforce safety, satisfaction, productivity and energy efficiency?

Traditionally, hospital leaders have asked five questions when considering a major building project:

1. Urgency – Is the expansion/replacement actually needed now to fulfill the hospital's mission? What is the cost strategically of not proceeding?
2. Appropriateness – Is the proposed plan the most reasonable and prudent in relation to other alternatives?
3. Cost – Is the cost per square foot appropriate in relation to other projects in the region?
4. Financial impact – Has the financial impact of additional volume, depreciation expense and revenue assumptions been reasonably analyzed and projected?
5. Sources of funds – Is the anticipated combination of additional operating income, reserves, borrowing and philanthropy reasonable and adequate to support the project?

Today, hospital leaders should also address a sixth question:

6. Evidence-based design – Will the proposed project incorporate all the relevant and proven evidence-based design innovations in order to optimize patient safety, quality and satisfaction as well as workforce safety, satisfaction, productivity and energy efficiency?

From questions to action: Ten steps to implement evidence-based design (including the business case)

To address question six effectively, a hospital should undertake at least the following 10 steps:

1. Create a multidisciplinary leadership team and develop a compelling vision to achieve measurable safety/quality improvements involving patients, families and staff, as well as volume and the bottom line.
2. Select an architect with proven understanding and experience in evidence-based design. Ask for specific examples of planned or completed projects where the firm was instrumental in assuring that evidence-based design innovations were included and implemented. Look for architects that are Evidence-based Design Assessment and Certification (EDAC) certified.
3. Identify evidence-based design interventions. Management, medical staff and board leadership must collaborate with the architects to determine which cost effective, evidence-based design interventions will support their vision for the new project.
4. Evaluate current practice and develop a baseline. For example, determine the current rates of infections, transfers, employee turn over, patient falls institutionally and at the patient unit level. Identify the baseline operating costs associated with these outcomes.
5. Set measurable post-occupancy improvement targets. For example, identify a reduction in hospital-acquired infections from X to Y; an increase in patient satisfaction rates from A to B; a decrease in workforce lift injuries from C to D; and reduction in patient transfers from E to F. These measurable improvement targets must be agreed to by all key stakeholders and widely communicated. Key staff members must be included

in this process and become active advocates. To be successful, it is essential to build an organizational culture of support for these changes.

6. Incorporate design improvements into capital and operating budgets. Management and medical leadership must incorporate the financial impact of these improvements into the hospital's annual capital and operating budgets to be reviewed and approved by the board of trustees.

7. Widely communicate improvement targets. Performance improvement targets should be included in all appropriate internal and external communications, including the methods used to collect data. This can provide public awareness and recognition that can differentiate the organization in the market place and increase market share.

8. Track and report progress. Upon completion of the new facility or renovation, the metrics of impact (including financial impact) at the overall institutional level and the unit level should be regularly reported to all key stakeholders, including the board.

9. Continually, incorporate new evidence-based design strategies. Regularly, review internal experience and new developments in evidence-based design research. Where appropriate, incorporate new evidence-based design interventions into the organization's facility maintenance activities, process and culture. While tracking results should continue for at least three years post-occupancy, new environmental design and process improvements should be systematically incorporated.

10. Publish your results. The organization should share lessons learned and publish its results (including financial results) with the rest of the health care and design communities. This will contribute to needed knowledge about the financial and clinical impact of evidence-based design.

(REFERENCE: This analysis is drawn from the article by Sadler, DuBose, & Zimring, "The Business Case for Building Better Hospitals Through Evidence Based Design," *Health Environments Research and Design Journal*, June 2008.)

CONCLUSION

Hospital leaders and boards of trustees face a new reality: they can no longer tolerate preventable hospital-acquired conditions such as infections and falls; injuries to staff; unnecessary intra-hospital patient transfers that can increase errors; or subjecting patients and families to noisy, confusing environments that increase anxiety and stress. They must effectively deploy all reasonable quality improvement techniques available. To be optimally effective, techniques will almost always rely on tactics that, when implemented, will produce best results.

Leaders must understand the clear connection between constructing well designed healing environments and improved health care safety and quality for patients, families and staff, as well as the compelling business case for doing so. The physical environment in which people work and patients receive their care is one of the essential elements to address a number of preventable hospital acquired conditions.

Emerging pay for performance methodologies that reward hospitals for quality and refuse to pay hospitals for harm they cause further strengthen the business case. At the same time that the costs of unnecessary harm are increasing, public and employer expectations are growing. The emerging practice of not charging for errors and the public reporting of comparable patient satisfaction scores add more weight to the revenue side of the business case. While much of the reimbursement and transparent public reporting requirements have been driven by Medicare, children's hospital leaders should take them into account as Medicaid and commercial payers adopt the same or similar practices.

As part of their management and fiduciary responsibilities, hospital leaders and boards must include cost effective evidence-based design interventions in all programs or risk economic consequences in an increasingly competitive and transparent environment. Implemented successfully, responsible use of evidence-based design will improve patient safety and quality, enhance workforce recruitment and retention and produce a significant multi-year return on investment. The effectiveness of any evidence-based design interventions will not occur in isolation from other process improvements that must be implemented concurrently. Similar to the experience of Institute for Healthcare Improvement in the 100,000 Lives and 5 Million Lives campaigns, effective change packages are a bundle of improvements that must be implemented together. The key point is that environmental design innovations included here are essential ingredients in optimally improving safety and quality.

As hospital leaders undertake building projects, it is imperative that they track ongoing operating savings as an integral part of their analyses. Hospital boards and management must hold each other accountable to new levels of environmental excellence and efficiency. Building a new hospital or undertaking a major renovation is likely to be the biggest financial decision that a board will ever make. It also provides a unique opportunity to transform the culture and processes of the overall organizational enterprise to maximize the investment. Hospital leaders have an opportunity and an obligation to assure that whether patients are in their care for an hour, a day, a week or a year, they are provided an optimal healing environment.

EXECUTIVE SUMMARY | 17

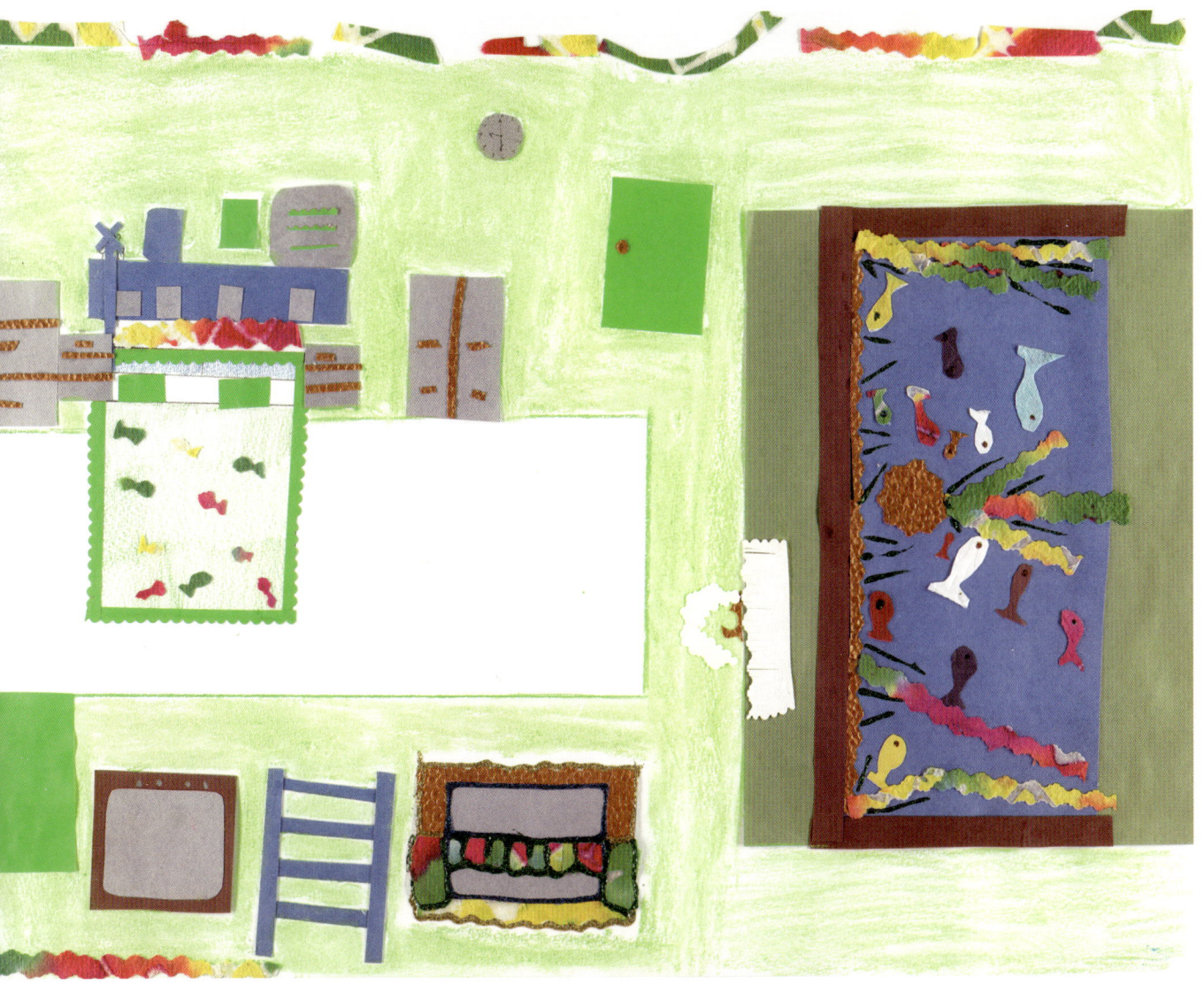

The Ideal Patient Room, Visual art, collage
Artwork by Nancy Hernandez (Nancy died in May 2005 at age 10.)
Children's National Medical Center, Washington, DC

3 | TRANSFORMING CARE IN CHILDREN'S HOSPITALS THROUGH ENVIRONMENTAL DESIGN

Literature Review

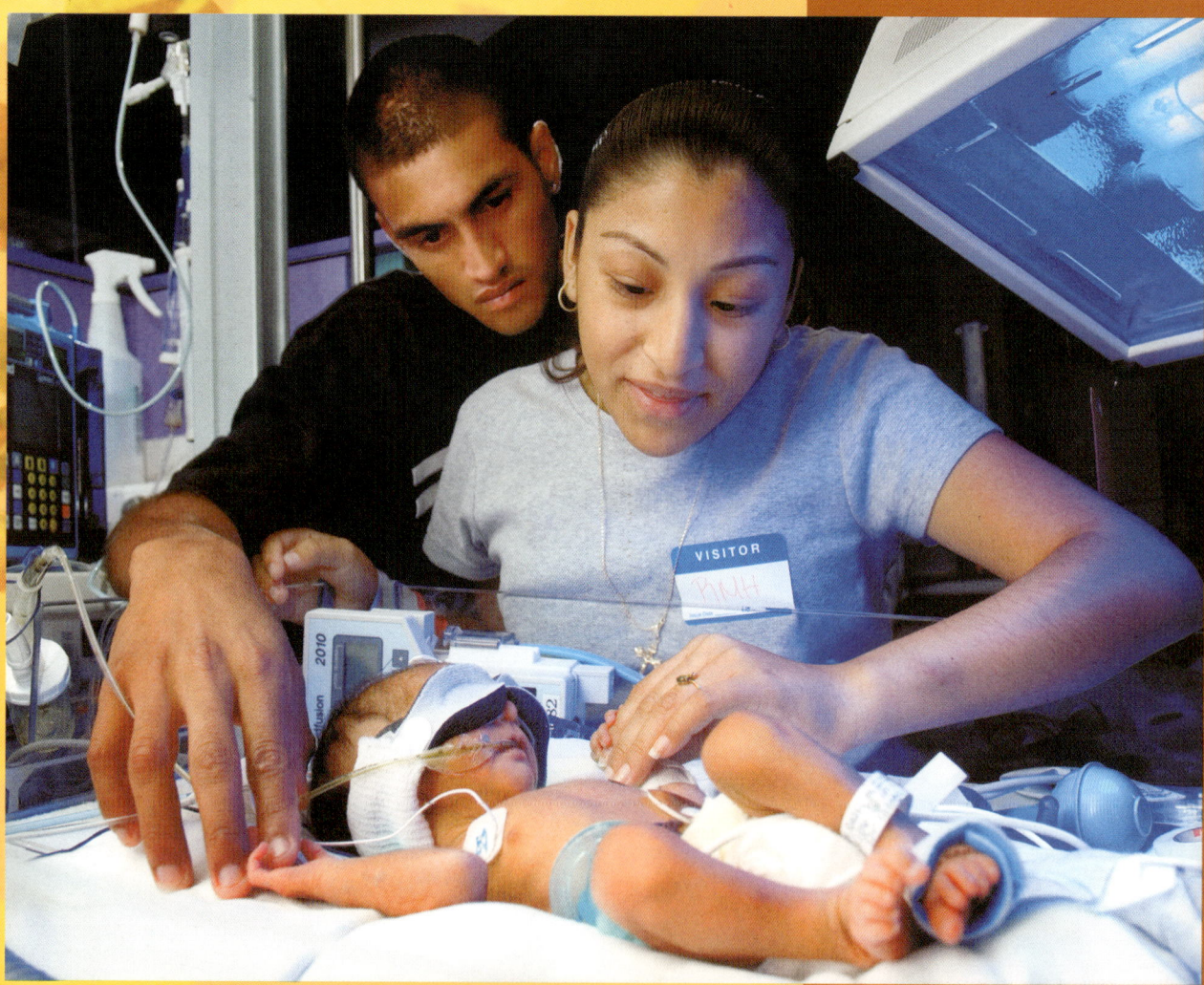

Parents Daisy Lopez and Alvaro Rodriguez wait patiently while their newborn daughter Natalie Rodriguez receives treatment for jaundice under an ultraviolet light.
photo by Allen S. Kramer, Texas Children's Hospital, Houston, TX

THE CENTER FOR HEALTH DESIGN

ANJALI JOSEPH, Ph.D.
Director of Research

AMY KELLER, M. Arch
Research Associate

KATIE KRONICK
Project Manager

> A hospital is a human invention and, as such can be changed at anytime.
> —Leland Kaiser

We are currently in the midst of an unprecedented building boom in the health care industry with some $100 billion in inflation-adjusted dollars spent on new hospital construction in the past five years (Henriksen, Isaacson, Sadler, & Zimring, 2007). Children's hospitals are following this trend to upgrade, expand, replace existing facilities or build new ones. The key drivers for this include aging of existing facilities (built in 1950s-1960s), advances in treating childhood diseases, technological advances, growing importance of patient centered and family centered care and a focus on advancing patient safety. Further, current health care settings are extremely inadequate and inefficient for the work practices and technologies that have evolved over the last 50 years. The Institute of Medicine in its 2001 report *Crossing the Quality Chasm* identified problems with the health care system in the United States deeming it unsafe, ineffective, inefficient, untimely, inequitable and lacking patient centeredness. A growing body of research shows that the physical design of health care settings contributes to these negative outcomes experienced so frequently in health care. On the other hand, thoughtful evidence-based facility design can help bring the patient, staff and families into the center of the health care experience; increase patient safety in the health care environment; and advance the overall quality of care provided. It is imperative to rethink facility design as a critical element in bringing about change in the way health care is provided and experienced especially in children's health care settings.

Two previous publications have addressed the literature associated with the research and design of pediatric facilities, both published under the auspices of the now defunct Association for the Care of Children's Health (Olds & Daniel, 1987; Shepley, Fournier, & McDougal, 1998). More recently, in-depth literature reviews conducted by different researchers in the last four years have identified a large and growing body of research linking the physical design of health care facilities with patient and staff outcomes (Chaudhury, Mahmood, & Valente, 2003; Joseph, 2006a, 2006b, 2007; Joseph & Ulrich, 2007; R. S. Ulrich, Zimring, Joseph, Quan, & Chaudhury, 2004). However, the focus of these literature reviews was primarily on adult acute care settings. Children's care environments are different in many ways from adult care environments: children have different developmental, psychosocial and physical needs from adults and the family plays a decision making role in the care process. Further, other issues such as providing opportunities for play, education and peer support may not be addressed in literature reviews focused on adult settings. On the other hand, some issues related to advancing patient safety, reducing medical errors and increasing staff effectiveness might be relevant in adult as well as pediatric settings.

The purpose of *Evidence for Innovation* is to systematically review the scientific literature that specifically concentrates on the relationship between environmental design and outcomes for patients, staff and families within children's health care settings. Findings from research in adult settings that are likely relevant in pediatric settings are also discussed briefly. Three key domains within the role of the physical environment are examined here:
- Advancing patient centered and family centered care
- Promoting safety
- Increasing staff effectiveness in providing care

STUDY METHODOLOGY

The purpose of this study was twofold:
- To provide an overview of the literature linking the design of the physical environment with outcomes in pediatric settings
- To identify gaps in this literature

A literature review was conducted to identify research studies on the impact of the physical environment on outcomes in pediatric health care settings including acute care, ambulatory care and long term care. Several online databases such as EBSCOhost, ProQuest, CINAHLdirect, PubMed, PsycINFO and Google Scholar were used to search for journal articles. In addition, the Center for Health Design database was searched to identify articles relevant to this study.

Combinations of keywords used to conduct advanced searches for articles include pediatric, children, neonatal, adolescent/teen, family, staff, neonatal intensive care unit (NICU), pediatric intensive care unit (PICU), hospitals, clinics, outpatient, design, environment, physical environment, family centered care, light, daylight, noise, nature, music, art, air quality, high efficiency particulate air (HEPA) filters, nursing station, single patient room, playroom, libraries, way finding, development, stress, infection, sleep, pain, agitation, patient safety, errors and satisfaction. The initial search yielded approximately 450 articles focused on pediatric settings. These include empirical studies as well as descriptive articles. Articles selected from this initial group met the following criteria:
- Published in peer-reviewed journals
- Empirical study or in-depth literature review conducted in a pediatric health care setting
- Clearly defined environmental variable

Approximately 320 articles met these criteria. Additionally, key literature reviews such as the 2004 literature review by Ulrich and colleagues. and other key studies conducted in adult health care settings that might be relevant to pediatric settings were included. These articles were assessed individually for quality, rigor and relevance to the study at hand. The studies were classified as one of the following types: experimental, quasi experimental, controlled observational (cohort or case control), observational (without control groups, surveys, case studies) and expert opinion. A majority of the studies identified were controlled observational or observational studies without control groups, or they were surveys or case studies. Within each of these categories, studies were rated as good, fair or poor using a set of established criteria. A sample of the selected studies was analyzed in detail. Refer to the appendix for further description of rating criteria and analysis of selected study samples.

CHILDREN IN HEALTH CARE ENVIRONMENTS

A child's lack of experience with hospital environments and situations can cause confusion, anxiety and fear. A child's loss of control over the small things that help him or her understand the world can lead to frustration. Separation from family and peers and not understanding the hospital visit add to the concern. The physical environment of the health care facility – whether inpatient or ambulatory – contributes to this fear and stress and impacts the healing process (R. S. Ulrich et al., 2004).

Designing children's care environments requires sensitivity. Key themes and issues especially relevant to children's environments provide the context for this report, including:

—*Varying needs of children in different age groups:* Children's needs vary considerably depending on age and developmental stage. Extremely fragile premature infants need protected and monitored environments. Even within the infant population, significant developmental differences exist (Shepley et al., 1998). Young children may find the hospital environment frightening, and the need for family support and presence is critical. Sick, but ambulatory, children need opportunities for play and stimulation. Adolescents may need privacy and personal space as well as socialization with peers and friends (A. Hutton, 2002). Children's different physical and psychosocial needs must be addressed through the design of the physical environment.

—*Role of the family:* Caregivers and families are integral to the care provided in children's health care environments. They participate in decision making and care giving, provide emotional and psychological support and aid the transition from hospital to home. For younger children especially, families are the link to the familiar. For older children, they provide support during a difficult period. While families and friends contribute to the well-being of a child in a health care setting, they, too, have great needs and fears. Studies show that encouraging family presence during difficult procedures and encouraging families to visit children at the bedside help to reduce anxiety among parents and caregivers and enable them to contribute constructively to care giving (Davidson et al., 2007).

Evidence for Innovation focuses on the role of the environment in promoting patient and family centered care, safety and effectiveness in children's health care settings. In each of these three influential areas, the specific needs of children will be addressed along with the role of the family.

ADVANCING PATIENT CENTERED AND FAMILY CENTERED CARE THROUGH DESIGN

The Institute for Family Centered Care defines patient and family centered care as an *"innovative approach to the planning, delivery, and evaluation of healthcare that is grounded in mutually beneficial partnerships among healthcare patients, families, and providers"* (The Institute for Family Centered Care, 2007). In patient and family centered care, all care options are tailored to the individual patient, and care giving activities revolve around providing comfort and emotional support to the patient with family and friends as active partners in the care process. Some core concepts are a willingness to understand and honor knowledge, values, beliefs and culture of the patient and family; communication of information openly between care providers and patients and families; and inclusion of patients and families in care and decision making (Henriksen et al. 2007; Saunders et al., 2003; Macnab, Thiessen, & Hinton, 2000).

While advancing patient centered and family centered care has become an important goal in any health care setting, this core concept guides program, policy and design in health care settings for children. In pediatric settings, parents and families play a central role, and studies show that involving family in a child's care has many potential benefits including: improved satisfaction with care, decreased parental stress, increased parental comfort and competence with post-discharge care, improved success with breastfeeding, shortened hospital lengths of stay, decreased readmissions and increased staff satisfaction (Forsythe, 1998; Meyer et al., 1994).

The physical environment is a core component of the care provided in children's health care settings and plays an important role in supporting the practice of patient and family centered care (Henriksen et al., 2007). Several studies show that physical environmental factors, such as noise, air quality, room layout, unit layout and availability of spaces for families, can impact sleep, stress, perception of pain and opportunities for families to spend time with their children (Ackerman, Sherwonit, & Fisk, 1989; Bellieni et al., 2003; Shepley et al., 1998; L. K. Zahr, & de Traversay, 1995). An environment focused more on treating the disease rather than caring for the patient will be filled with cues such as smells, clutter of equipment, noise, that disengage patients and families from the healing process. Research studies show that environments can be designed with the patients and families at the core so the result is improved clinical and physiological outcomes for patients (Shepley et al., 1998). Thoughtfully designed children's care environments can support patients, families and staff psychologically by providing greater control, protecting confidentiality and privacy, and facilitating communication and participation in care.

Improving Clinical and Physiological Outcomes

Many aspects of the physical environment affect clinical and physiological outcomes among children. Studies show that environmental changes such as reducing noise levels, improving lighting, adding music and providing single bed rooms can influence outcomes such as sleep, medication use, stress, development and convalescence.

Impact of noise on sleep and developmental outcomes

Recommended noise levels for pediatric wards have been set as low as 45 db during the day, though decibel levels up to 72 db are common (Couper et al., 1994). Noise in the PICUs has a number of related causes: visitation, open bay wards, equipment and equipment alarms, and staff conversations (R. Berens, 1999; Couper et al., 1994).

The high noise levels in children's hospitals significantly impact clinical outcomes, especially sleep. Patients in the PICU sleep significantly less than is normal for children of the same ages, and their patterns of sleep are seriously disturbed due to high noise levels and disturbance by staff (Al-Samsam & Cullen, 2005; Cureton-Lane & Fontaine, 1997). In addition, ICU patients spend significantly less time in REM (rapid eye movement) state than healthy children, and they suffer from hearing loss (R. Berens, 1999). In a prospective observational study of mechanically ventilated PICU patients, severe alterations to sleep patterns over a 24-hour period were linked to high noise levels (consistently higher than 48 db) and frequent staff interruptions. The researchers found that active sleep was reduced to a mere 3 percent of total sleep time. Sleep was highly fragmented with patients waking up an average of 40 times (Al-Samsam & Cullen, 2005). Further, sudden loud noises over and above ambient noise were linked to number of awakenings among infants. If the noise levels remain high (over 76 db – typical hospital nursery noise), infants are not likely to adjust to the noise and will not be able to go back to sleep (Philbin & Klaas, 2000).

The research on noise reducing environmental interventions for pediatric intensive care units has been sparse. A study conducted in an open bay infant ward and an open bay pediatric ward found that a high number of people moving through the open wards resulted in high noise levels. This was particularly true on weekends. The research suggests abolishing open wards and establishing control measures to reduce noise levels (Couper et al., 1994). Ulrich and colleagues (2004) in a literature review on the impact of the physical environment on outcomes in acute care settings suggest that single occupancy rooms with closed doors would help in reducing noise levels at the patient's bedside since roommates and families are often the source of disturbances.

Much of the research on noise in children's hospital environments has been conducted in NICUs and nurseries. Noise poses critical concerns in such environments. Premature infants are among the most vulnerable and at-risk patients, requiring the most vigilant care and machines. The presence of many staff, family members and mechanical equipment make the NICU a noisy place.

The Committee to Establish Recommended Standards for Newborn ICU Design recommends that noise not exceed a continuous sound level pressure (Leq) of 45 db, that sound level pressure is not greater than 50 db 10 percent of the time during each hour (L10), and that transient sounds (Lmax) are no greater than 65 db (White & Dunn, 2006). Unfortunately, numerous studies demonstrate that many NICUs exceed these recommended standards (Byers, Waugh, & Lowman, 2006; Chang, Lin, & Lin, 2001; Kent, Tan, Clarke, & Bardell, 2002; Lawson, Daum, & Turkewitz, 1977; Levy, Woolston, & Browne, 2003). One study measured both the Leq and L10 at 60 db (Byers et al., 2006). These results are typical of study findings. The high noise levels to which infants are exposed can have detrimental effects, both in the short term as well as in long-term development and wellness. Infants exposed to excessive noise levels in the NICU have been shown to have poor auditory system development, auditory attention and stress (R. Berens, 1999; Bremmer, Byers, & Kiehl, 2003; Gray & Philbin, 2005).

Many studies show that interventions to reduce noise levels can be extremely beneficial to infants in NICUs and nurseries. Altering noise levels in the incubator can efficiently alter the environment and does not require facility renovations. Placing earmuffs on the infants, covering the incubator, installing a sound absorbing panel in the incubator, and putting sound absorbing foam next to the infant have all demonstrated physiological benefits for infant development and convalescence (Bellieni et al., 2003; Johnson, 2001; Saunders, 1995; Zahr & de Traversay, 1995). Some of these interventions have been shown to decrease heart rate, decrease respiratory rate, increase time spent in regular sleep, decrease sleep/awake state changes and increase oxygen saturation (Johnson, 2001; Zahr & de Traversay, 1995).

Comprehensive interventions targeting multiple changes simultaneously have also proven effective. One hospital implemented education session on the negative effects of noise in the NICU, installed noise indicator lights near nurses work stations, implemented a quiet hour, readjusted the feeding schedule in accordance with infant wake patterns, instructed parents about noise and structurally reduced the noise admitted by a set of doors. The significant noise reductions achieved through these interventions remained constant through the first 12 months after implementation (Thear & Wittmann-Price, 2006). In another study, noise reductions were achieved through the implementation of a one-hour quiet period. The reduced noise levels were associated with improved outcomes among the infants, including decreased blood pressure, decreased arterial pressure and less infant activity (Slevin, Farrington, Duffy, Daly, & Murphy, 2000).

In addition to equipment and targeted alterations, complete or partial renovations can also decrease noise. Materials substitution and equipment placement can decrease noise exposure for infants. During construction of a developmental NICU, one hospital included sound-absorbing flooring, wall panels, ceiling tiles and privacy curtains (Byers et al., 2006). In that same study, researchers looked at the impact of new and more advanced equipment on noise levels. Researchers found that renovations and new equipment resulted in significant decreases in the noise level (Byers et al., 2006). An additional study found that modifying the sound environment by installing weather stripping, replacing metal trash cans with rubber ones, covering incubators, installing carpet and installing sound-absorbing material throughout the bay significantly reduced noise without any risk to patient safety (Walsh, Reitenbach, Hudson, & DePompei, 2001). Berens and Weigle (1996) conducted a cost-benefit analysis of installing sound absorbing ceiling tiles in an open bay NICU. The mean noise levels reduced from 55 db to 53 db after renovations. The researchers did not measure the impact on reverberation times (long reverberation times indicate "building up" of sound that impacts perceived noise levels and sound quality). A study conducted in an adult coronary critical care unit found that high performance sound absorbing acoustical ceiling tiles helped to improve the environment by reducing noise and reverberation (Blomkvist, Eriksen, Theorell, Ulrich, & Rasmanis, 2005). This type of intervention likely relates to pediatric settings as well.

Clearly, research has concentrated more on the effects of noise on infants as compared to general pediatric patient groups. Yet still more studies are needed on the effects of noise as well as design interventions on outcomes among children and adolescents in health care settings. Further, more research is needed to demonstrate the long-term effectiveness of these interventions as well as the long-term negative effects of loud noise in the NICU.

Impact of lighting on developmental outcomes

Several studies show that infants are sensitive to light exposure and that the environment of the NICU impacts physiological outcomes and visual development among preterm infants (Graven, 2004). No studies were identified that looked at hospitalized young children or adolescents.

Studies suggest that exposure to light is an effective treatment for neonatal hyperbilirubinaemia (neonatal jaundice) (Giunta & Rath, 1969). This disorder is common to premature infants who lack the ability to metabolize bilirubin, a product of the decomposition of hemoglobin in dead red blood cells (McColl & Veitch, 2001). Exposure to light bleaches the bilirubin into a form that can be excreted from the body. In a controlled study of 96 preterm infants, 47 unclothed (except for diapers) babies were exposed to bright light (90 footcandles), and 49 fully clothed babies, to dim light (10 footcandles). The group of infants exposed to bright light showed lower serum bilirubin as compared to the infants who were exposed to dim light (Giunta & Rath, 1969).

One potential negative result of overexposure to light in health care settings is retinal damage in preterm infants, and a few studies suggest that reducing ambient lighting in hospital nurseries might improve outcomes (Ackerman et al., 1989; Mann, Haddow, Stokes, Goodley, & Rutter, 1986). Neonatal infants have thinner eyelids and usually have not developed the ability to constrict their pupils in response to light exposure. High intensity illumination in their environment makes them susceptible to retinal damage. However, studies examining the impact of reduced ambient lighting on retinopathy among premature infants have failed to detect a causal link (Kennedy et al., 2001; Reynolds, Hardy, Kennedy, & Spencer, 1998; Seiberth, Linderkamp, Knorz, & Liesenhoff, 1994).

Four studies show that providing cycled lighting (reduced light levels at night) in NICUs results in improved sleep and weight gain among preterm infants (Blackburn & Patteson, 1991; Brandon, Holditch-Davis, & Belyea, 2002; Mann et al., 1986; C. L. Miller, White, Whitman, O'Callaghan, & Maxwell, 1995). In one study, 41 preterm infants in structurally identical critical care units were provided either cycled lighting or constant light levels during the day and night during a lengthy hospital stay. Compared to infants with constant light levels, infants assigned to the cycled lighting had a greater rate of weight gain, were able to be fed orally sooner, spent fewer days on the ventilator and on phototherapy, and displayed enhanced motor coordination (C. L. Miller et al., 1995).

Most of the studies examining the impact of light – natural or artificial – have been conducted in NICU settings. There are no known studies examining how exposure to light might impact older hospitalized children. Studies conducted among hospitalized adults show that exposure to light helps in reducing depression, intake of pain medication and length of stay (Beauchemin & Hays, 1996; Benedetti, Colombo, Barbini, Campori, & Smeraldi, 2001; Walch et al., 2005). Exposure to light might have similar benefits for children as well, but additional research is needed in this area.

Impact of the environment on stress

The hospital experience is extremely stressful for children who face being away from family, entering an unfamiliar environment and the anticipating of painful procedures. Patients also experience stress directly related to medical procedures such as Computed Tomography (CT) scans, which often require sedation. Finally, the stress related to pain and painful procedures often exacerbates the patient's perception of pain. Though none of these stressors can be eliminated from the experience of a child needing acute care, interventions within the physical environment can greatly augment the child or infant's experience and reduce stress, pain perception and medication use.

The environment in which a patient is hospitalized should be conducive to his or her wellness experience, not add to fears. Nurses say they often use background noise, such as music, and create a familiar environment to increase the comfort level of their patients (Polkki, Vehvilainen, & Pietla, 2001). Music can decrease the anxiety and stress level of patients even when used as background noise. Music is effective at decreasing anxiety both in preparing for the procedure and during the procedure phases (Brice & Barclay, 2007). Studies conducted among children have found that recorded lullabies are an effective distraction in reducing overall distress in children receiving routine immunizations (Malone, 1996; Megel, Houser, & Gleaves, 1998).

Exposure to nature – viewing the garden, gardening, sitting in the garden – have all demonstrated a calming and restorative effect for many populations. Gardens in children's health care settings are a place where children, their families and staff can get away to play or to meditate. A study was conducted on the perceptions of families and staff regarding the benefits of a garden in a pediatric hospital in Malaysia (Said, Salleh, Abu Bakar, & Mohamad, 2005). Parents felt that spending time in the garden was extremely beneficial to their children. Some perceived benefits included increased independence among children, reduced emotional disturbances, increased cheerful and agile behaviors, increased cooperative and obedient behavior, decreased emotional distress, and increased feelings of wellness (Said, 2003; Said & Abu Bakar, 2004). Exposure to gardens has potentially beneficial effects on emotional states, feelings of anxiety, sadness, anger, worry and pain (Sherman, Varni, Ulrich, & Malcarne, 2005). Most studies conducted on the impact of gardens are observational or based on perception. Additional rigorous research is needed to examine the impact of gardens on objective measures of stress.

Stress related outcomes in the NICU are often inextricably intertwined with developmental outcomes. Infants show preference to human speech, especially their mothers' voices, and music, and exposure to such sounds has been linked to auditory development and learning among infants (Philbin & Klaas, 2000). Studies show that music can be an effective way to decrease infant stress. Music is shown to increase oxygen saturation levels, decrease heart rate, decrease behavioral issues and decrease the incidence of respiratory pause (Arnon et al., 2006; Shepley, 2006). One study compared the effects of live music, recorded music, no music on preterm infants' heart rates, respiratory rates, sleep/awake states, and oxygen saturation levels. While the effects on the infants during the live music therapy were not significant, 30 minutes after the live music therapy, there were significant decreases in heart rate and sleep/awake measurements when compared with both no therapy and recorded music groups (Arnon et al., 2006).

Most hospitals are extremely confusing, and the experience of finding the way in these complex settings is extremely stressful for patients, families and visitors. In a study conducted at a major regional 604-bed tertiary care hospital, the annual cost of the way finding system was calculated at more than $220,000 per year in the main hospital or $448 per bed per year in 1990. Much of this cost was hidden when directions were given by people other than information staff; this consumed more than 4,500 staff hours, the equivalent of more than two full-time positions (Zimring, 1990). Most studies on the impact of physical environment on way finding have been conducted in adult health care settings, but way finding problems are not unique to adult settings (Carpman & Grant, 1993). A good way finding system includes four main components that work at different levels: administrative and procedural (mail maps and hospital pre-visit information); external building cues (signage and location of parking); local information (you-are-here maps, signage at key decision points, directories, clear nomenclature); and global structure (simple and accessible building layout) (R. S. Ulrich et al., 2004). The findings from adult settings can likely be applied to way finding systems in pediatric settings although additional consideration should be given to child friendly signage and cues.

Impact of the environment on perception of pain and medication use

Pain is often an unavoidable aspect of the hospital experience. Whether pain is continuous or specific to a procedure, many children endure painful hospital moments. Necessarily, a lot of attention is paid to ways this pain can be alleviated. Due to the risks often involved with sedatives and pain medications, researchers are looking at non-pharmacological methods for reducing pain in children. Studies on the usefulness of sedatives in children have shown that drug overdoses and negative interactions between drugs are the most frequent causes of negative outcomes (Cote, Karl, Notterman, Weinberg, & McCloskey, 2000). Furthermore, not only are sedatives often dangerous, but they also can be ineffective for older children (Greenberg, Faeber, Aspinall, & Adams, 1993). Interventions in the physical environment can be beneficial both for patients undergoing procedures under sedation and for patients enduring painful procedures while awake.

In order to decrease the use of sedatives during procedures, music therapy can be a highly effective for inducing sleep in patients. One study on the effectiveness of music therapy during non-invasive procedures found that it was effective for 100 percent of ECG (electrocardiogram) patients, 80.7 percent of CT scan patients, and 94.1 percent of other procedure patients in inducing a sleep state without sedation (Walworth, 2005). Furthermore, a cost analysis for this study found that music therapy saved money, time, staff resources and equipment resources. Additionally, even when compared with a sedative, music therapy is more effective and efficient; patients receiving music therapy fell asleep more quickly and did not have any of the negative effects of the sedative such as difficulty returning to an awake state (Loewy, Hallan, Friedman, & Martinez, 2005).

During painful procedures, music therapy can also decrease a patient's perception of pain. Music before and after invasive procedures, such as needle sticks, distracts the child, decreasing his or her observable distress. However, children who are distracted in the pre-procedure phase show more intense distress during the actual procedure, but the duration is shorter. The surprise of the needle stick increases the initial perception of pain, while decreasing the length of time the pain is felt (Malone, 1996).

Developments in new technology also have made painful procedures easier for children to endure. Virtual reality games and programs have been used during painful procedures to decrease pain perception. Several studies have examined the effectiveness of virtual reality distractions among pediatric oncology patients undergoing painful procedures such as chemotherapy (Gershon, Zimand, Lemos, Rothbaum, & Hodges, 2003; Hoffman, Doctor, Patterson, Carrougher, & Furness, 2000; Schneider & Workman, 1999; Wolitzky, Fivush, Zimand, Hodges, & Rothbaum, 2005). Such interventions have shown to be effective in reducing pain and anxiety and symptom distress. These programs are not only effective for patients receiving a procedure for the first time, but also for children, such as oncology patients, who experience recurring painful procedures (Malone, 1996; Wolitzky et al., 2005). One study showed that virtual reality games used in conjunction with opioid treatment for burn care patients helped to reduce pain experienced and served as a nonpharmacologic analgesic (Hoffman et al., 2000).

For stress and pain management and medication use, nonpharmacological approaches to treatment are essential. Though significant research demonstrates the positive effects of interventions such as music, additional research is needed to determine the effectiveness on stress and perception of pain when patients view artwork or nature from their rooms. Positive distractions should not only be seen as a way to improve psychological experiences, but physiological and clinical experiences as well.

Improving Clinical and Physiological Outcomes – Summary and Recommendations

The fragile state of the patients in the NICU makes them especially vulnerable to the harmful effects of environmental factors such as loud noise, high light levels and infectious pathogens. Exposure to excessive noise in the NICU impacts short-term and long-term auditory development. Removing sources of loud noises, instituting quiet hours, educating staff and parents, and providing closed bays (instead of open wards) are effective in reducing noise. Sound absorbing acoustical ceiling tiles are also effective in reducing noise and reverberation. Additionally, the following have demonstrated physiological benefits for infant development and convalescence: placing earmuffs on the infant, covering the incubator, installing a sound absorbing panel in the incubator and putting sound absorbing foam next to the infant.

Loud noises are common in general pediatric settings as well and strategies such as providing closed bays and closing room doors have shown to be effective in reducing noise levels. Few studies have examined how noise impacts young children, adolescents or families on pediatric units.

Cycled lighting (reduced light levels at night) and providing focused lighting over incubators helped to improve sleep and developmental outcomes among infants. Light is also beneficial in treating neonatal jaundice. Many new NICU designs are moving from open wards to single patient rooms with the primary purpose of providing an environment that can be customized to the developmental and health needs of the infant. Studies suggest that families and staff are also more satisfied in these environments.

Studies conducted in inpatient and outpatient settings show that distractions such as virtual reality can help in reducing anxiety, distress and perceived pain associated with difficult procedures. Music and music therapy is also an effective intervention in reducing stress and anxiety and reducing pain and need for sedation among hospitalized and ambulatory patients. Spending time in gardens is also effective in improving mood, reducing distress and increasing feelings of wellness among young children. Other studies show that the physical environment can promote healing among children. Room design and ambience and use of music help patients cope with pain and aggression.

Key recommendations include:
- Install high performance sound absorbing ceiling tiles
- Incorporate music as a positive distraction during procedures
- Use virtual reality games and artwork as positive distractions
- Install incubator noise reduction measures in the NICU
- Practice circadian (cycled) lighting in the NICU
- Improve signage and cues to ease way finding
- Conduct a noise audit
- Incorporate accessible gardens
- Optimize natural light in staff and patient areas

Improving Psychosocial Outcomes

An important aspect of patient and family centered care is providing comfort and emotional support to patients and families and empowering them to become participants in the care giving process. Research studies show that many psychosocial outcomes central to promoting patient and family centered care can be improved through the design of the physical environment. These include improving coping skills, encouraging opportunities for play and education, increasing privacy and control, enhancing way finding, and increasing satisfaction.

Improving coping skills

Frequent or prolonged hospitalization may negatively impact children's psychological well-being and increase the risk for long term emotional and behavioral difficulties. To combat the risk of emotional, behavioral and developmental troubles, investing in the mental well-being of a child should be a priority. Environmental design strategies can be effective in helping a child cope with illness and anxiety or fear of the hospital visit (Boyd & Hunsberger, 1998). A child's ability to cope with illness is enhanced by familiarity with the environment and presence of supportive caregivers as well as advance knowledge of upcoming procedures.

To help a child cope with his/her hospital experience, family members can provide distraction, emotional and verbal expression, independent activities, familiarity, and knowledge (Bers, Gonzalez-Heydrich, & DeMaso, 2003; Boyd & Hunsberger, 1998; Davidson et al., 2007; Junior, Coutinho, & Ferreira, 2006; Robb, 2000). Providing ample family space in each patient room to encourage parents and siblings to remain with the child can result in ongoing support (Boyd & Hunsberger, 1998). Activities such as televisions, computers, virtual reality games and quiet rooms can help with coping by providing distractions from pain and anxiety (Junior et al., 2006).

One study explored using a kaleidoscope as a distraction for reducing pain in needle-stick procedures. The experimental group who used the kaleidoscope perceived less pain and demonstrated less behavioral distress than the control group who did not use the kaleidoscope (Vessey, Carlson, & McGill, 1994). Two studies found that using virtual reality as a distraction during painful procedures in outpatient pediatric oncology clinics resulted in lower pain and anxiety ratings, reduced pulse, and reduced behavioral distress (Gershon et al., 2003; Wolitzky et al., 2005). Studies previously described show that music is also an effective intervention in calming pediatric patients and enabling them to cope with pain.

Room design and ambience may help in calming agitated or aggressive hospitalized children. In one study, standard quiet rooms were compared to an altered room (Colored paint was added to white walls, vinyl floor was carpeted; and a mural was painted on one wall.) to test whether or not the more attractive environment resulted in patients becoming calmer faster. Total aggression ratings were 45 percent lower in the modified quiet room than in the standard quiet room; initial aggression scores fell by 50 percent during five minutes in the modified quiet room, but only after 20 minutes in the standard quiet room (Glod et al., 1994).

Viewing artwork depicting images of nature has been linked with stress reduction for diverse groups of people. Studies conducted among adult patients show that viewing nature images such as water, trees or high depth of field results in reduced anxiety and pain (R. S. Ulrich & Gilpin, 2003). A preliminary study conducted with children and their siblings in a pediatric emergency department suggests that interactive art cart programs help in substantially reducing their fear and anxiety. Of the 61 children surveyed, 92 percent said that the program helped them forget their fear, concern or anxiety (K. McDonald, 2006). This is a low cost intervention that can be incorporated into any pediatric facility.

Providing social support
The importance of maintaining links to familiar environments, routines and activities cannot be underestimated in the care of hospitalized children. This might include providing opportunities for children to interact with friends in their regular school classrooms or with peers who are also hospitalized. This is particularly important for adolescent patients (A. Hutton, 2002, 2003). Several studies mention that contact with peers results in significant benefits in social and communication skills and in the development of greater self-confidence and independence among pediatric patients (Fels, Waalen, Zhai, & Weiss, 2001; Said & Abu Bakar, 2004; Said et al., 2005).

The computerized network, Starbright World was created to link seriously ill children to an interactive online virtual community that enables them to play games, talk about their illnesses or learn about their conditions along with other chronically ill children. Since the inception of the Starlight Starbright programs, several research studies have shown improved outcomes: reduction in pain and distress, reduction in the fear and isolation of a prolonged illness, greater willingness to return for treatment, increased sense of peer support, increased knowledge and sense of responsibility for managing disease, distraction from the challenges that accompany their illness, and increased ability to cope with their diseases (Battles & Wiener, 2002; Brokstein, Cohen, & Walco, 2002; Bush, Huchital, & Simonian, 2002; Holden, Bearison, Rode, Fishman, & Rosenberg, 2001; Holden, Bearison, Rode, Rosenberg, & Fishman, 1999; Rode, Capitulo, Fishman, & Holden, 1998). An experimental research study evaluated the impact of the Starbright World on children's pain, mood, loneliness and willingness to return for treatment in an outpatient setting. Children ages 8-19 years who were HIV infected or had a life-threatening illness were the focus of the study. The children spent an average of one hour or less per month using the Starbright World. The findings revealed that 33 percent of the children were more willing to return to the hospital for treatment; 52 percent of the children felt decreases in loneliness; and 24 percent reported that the Starbright World helped with depressed mood and increases in energetic mood (Battles & Wiener, 2002).

A study linking children in a hospital with their regular school classrooms combined video conferencing with robotics. The concentration, initiative and communication interactions of remote students were measured. Over time, the remote students were able to engage in the same tasks as their peers, initiate positive contributions to the classrooms and communicate ideas (Fels et al., 2001). Interventions such as these have great potential to improve the hospital experience for children by helping them stay connected to their peers (Battles & Wiener, 2002; Bers, Gonzalez-Heydrich, Raches, & DeMaso, 2001; Rassine, Gutman, & Silner, 2004).

Encouraging opportunities for play and education
Play is an integral part of a child's life. A child who plays has fun, develops courage, imagination, resourcefulness, initiative, daring and an ability to cope in competitive situations (Haiat, Bar-Mor, & Shochat, 2003). Play has been used as a therapeutic tool to reduce tension, anxiety, anger, frustration and conflict among pediatric patients; it provides a means for children to "play out" frightening, stressful or frustrating experiences (Carvalho & Begnis, 2006; Craddock, 2003; Gariepy & Howe, 2003; Haiat et al., 2003; Ispa, Barrett, & Yanghee, 1988; Junior et al., 2006; Naka, Senda, Tsuji, & Yata, 2002; Pass & Bolig, 1993; Urazoe, Senda, Tsuji, & Yata, 2001; J. Vessey & Mahon, 1990; Wishon & Brown, 1991). Theoretical and empirical

arguments suggest that play allows children to regain control over things when they have lost control (Carvalho & Begnis, 2006; Craddock, 2003; Gariepy & Howe, 2003; Haiat et al., 2003; Junior et al., 2006; Kapelaki et al., 2003; Naka et al., 2002; Pass & Bolig, 1993; Said & Abu Bakar, 2004; Said et al., 2005; Urazoe et al., 2001; Wishon & Brown, 1991). With thoughtful planning, children's play can constructively deal with concerns about separation from family, routine, unfamiliar hospital personnel and procedures, institutionalization, and temporary immobility (Piserchia, Bragg, & Alvarez, 1982). One study examines whether or not exposing children to medical equipment before a procedure reduces anxiety. The researchers found that fewer signs of anxiety are observed when children are exposed to the equipment beforehand (Ispa et al., 1988).

Variability in chronological and mental ages, disability and equipment needs should all be considered when designing play spaces. The design of a play space is particularly important for children with disabilities because environmental variables can affect a child's ability to play. An observational study at a children's rehabilitation hospital explored the layout of a play space with a toy closet where balls, books, cars, trucks, crayons, puzzles, a TV, stereo, pool table and a play kitchen were stored (Eisert, Kulka, & Moore, 1988). After the observation, interviews with the pediatric care providers were conducted to determine needs and suggestions for modifying the space. The study concluded that the following would be effective: control unnecessary sources of stimulation by creating a neutral background environment; decrease clutter and improve storage; encourage exploration and self-initiation by using color and variety to define areas and display toys to increase accessibility; and allow for individual differences in age and physical and mental abilities. Pre- and post-test observations and the data revealed that in the existing space, 30 percent of the child's time was spent in play, while in the modified space, 60 percent of the child's time was spent in play (Eisert et al., 1988). The physical setting can contribute to observed differences in play behaviors. Several studies found that children in a playroom engaged in more conversation and in other activities such as feeding the fish than children in the non-playroom settings (Clatworthy, 1981; Pass & Bolig, 1993; Vavili, 2000). In one study, a hospital equipped with a well structured play environment was compared to a hospital with a non-structured play environment. Researchers found that the structured setting influenced the types of interactions and the types of play children chose as compared to the non-structured setting (Pass & Bolig, 1993). Organized play requires certain types of settings, which should be an important direction for future research. Research is also needed to understand how different types of structured and non-structured settings might help achieve therapy goals for different pediatric populations.

Video games have potential as an educational tool for medically challenged adolescents. Computer games give children pleasure and expose them to experiential learning and can be a good method for presenting health education. As we learned, exposing children to medical equipment prior to a procedure can help with coping skills and encourage educational play; a computer game can serve as a buffer between a child and the frightening reality of surgery by presenting information about a procedure in less intimidating manner. "It exposes the child to the surgical experience in a stimulated and safe setting, which could lower the child's anxiety level and help mentally prepare him or her for surgery"(Rassine et al., 2004). Understanding the educational and play-like aspects of the ever evolving technology can help improve the health care experience and should be considered for future research.

Increasing privacy and control

In multiple studies on patients' preferences in hospital settings, the need for privacy as well as control over spaces is a recurring theme (Altimier, 2004; Batista-Miranda, Darbey, Kelly, & Baurer, 1995; Blumberg & Devlin, 2006; Gusella, Ward, & Butler, 1998; D. D. Harris, Shepley, White, Kolberg, & Harrell, 2006; Hutton, 2002; Hutton, 2005). One qualitative study shows that adolescents have definite opinions about what they want in a hospital environment (Hutton, 2002). Responses from the sample of healthy adolescents surveyed about space and privacy in the hospital show a need for privacy in the bedroom, in performing grooming activities and in using the telephone. Additionally, adolescents said that having control over the space they inhabit would alleviate their fears of being interrupted when they want to be alone (A. Hutton, 2002). An exploratory study to capture adolescents' expectations and experiences while in a hospital ward discovered that the adolescent patient prefers privacy in the bedrooms, however, space for companionship and camaraderie is also desired (Hutton, 2003). Additionally, findings from this study stress the importance of private bathrooms in patient rooms; adolescents felt embarrassed having to use a shared bathroom (Hutton, 2003). A survey conducted on adolescents' room preferences (shared bedroom or private bedroom) demonstrates that adolescents have varying preferences for rooming arrangements; 40 percent of surveyed patients preferred to be in a private room while approximately the same number preferred a roommate (N. O. Miller, Friedman, & Coupey, 1998).

Single patient rooms support individuality and are more conducive to family involvement. The single family room design in a NICU provides a controlled and safe environment for infants as well as privacy and the opportunity to personalize for families (D. D. Harris et al., 2006; White, 2003). Additional advantages of a single patient room design in the NICU are appropriate lighting, sound and level of care for each infant's particular developmental state (White, 2003). In one NICU, the benefits of shifting from a traditional open-bay neonatal intensive care nursery to a single-room model of care was explored from different perspectives. Privacy and increased opportunities in private rooms to encourage parents' participation and access to their infant were the deciding factors for selecting a single-room model of care (Bowie, Hall, Faulkner, & Anderson, 2003). Another facility transitioning from an open bay model to the single-room model of care experienced increased family satisfaction due to individual privacy. Furthermore, lighting, sound levels and the frequency of monitor alarms decreased in this environment (Schoenbeck, 2006). A recent multi-method study at 11 Level III NICUs compared environmental characteristics, patient medical outcomes and staff perceptions of the environments in different types of NICU settings – single family rooms, open bay, combination (single, double and multi-occupancy areas in the same unit) and double occupancy (D. D. Harris et al., 2006). The study found that NICUs with single family rooms were most effective in increasing parent privacy and presence, compliance with the Health Insurance Portability and Accountability Act, increasing staff satisfaction and reducing stress (D. D. Harris et al., 2006). Additionally, a literature review conducted by Ulrich and colleagues in 2004 shows multi-occupancy rooms are linked to increased nosocomial infections, increased stress from noise, reduced quality of care and reduced satisfaction. Documented benefits of private patient rooms include far less noise, better communication from staff to patients and from patients to staff, superior accommodation of family, and consistently higher satisfaction with overall quality of care.

Maximizing family visitation and participation in care

Several studies show that family involvement in care is beneficial to patients (Davidson et al., 2007; K. Dill, 2006; K. Dill & Gance-Cleveland, 2005; Dubbs, 2006; Eckle & MacLean, 2001; Franck & Callery, 2004; Gold, Gorenflo, Schwenk, & Bratton, 2006; Kissoon, 2006; Krug et al., 2006; Levine, 2006; Macnab, Thiessen, McLeod, & Hinton, 2000; Mangurten et al., 2006; Matincheck, 2006; Nibert & Ondrejka, 2005; O'Gorman, 2007; Perkins & Buchhalter, 2006; Powers & Rubenstein, 1999; Sacchetti, Paston, & Carraccio, 2005; Schoenbeck, 2006; Smith, Hefley, & Anand, 2007; White & Dunn, 2006; Ygge, Lindholm, & Arnetz, 2006). Guidelines were derived from more than 300 studies to support the involvement of family in the patient centered intensive care unit (Davidson et al., 2007). The environmental recommendations include: providing an area for spiritual support, maximizing staff education, ensuring family presence at rounds and resuscitation, and supplying family friendly signage and way finding capabilities. Several studies assessed visitation and behavior of siblings of newborns. The data suggest that sibling visitation is not likely to be harmful and might be beneficial to the patient and family (Davidson et al., 2007; Giacoia, Rutledge, & West, 1985; Griffin, 2003; Lewis et al., 1991; Moore, Coker, DuBuisson, Sweet, & Edwards, 2003; Pelander & Leino-Kilpi, 2004). Children who were allowed to visit showed less negative behavior and more knowledge about their ill siblings than children not allowed to visit (Davidson et al., 2007).

Increasing patient and family satisfaction

According to the 2004 National Survey on Consumers' Experiences with Patient Safety and Quality Information, 40 percent of Americans think the quality of health care has worsened in the last five years. Many expectations regarding the quality of care in pediatric settings relate to the nurse, nursing activities and the environment (Pelander & Leino-Kilpi, 2004). Children expect entertainment, education, service, physical treatment, respect and safety within their health care environment (A. Hutton, 2002; Pelander & Leino-Kilpi, 2004; Rollins, 2004).

Several studies describe children's expectations about the physical environment; in summary, the expectations included having patient rooms large enough to accommodate activities such as playing games with siblings, parents and caregivers; entertainment such as videos and interactive communication systems to pass the time; and privacy (Ayako, Mitsuru, Yoshitaka, & Tsutomu, 2002; Carney et al., 2003; A. Hutton, 2002; Kieffer & Vaughn, 1981). Adolescent patients require a balance between privacy and intimacy and social interaction with people (Mulhall, Kelly, & Pearce, 2004). Additionally, one study at an adolescent cancer center discovered that programmed amenities such as music or pool table helped to remove or reduce the feeling of being in a hospital and were preferred by adolescents and their families (Mulhall et al., 2004).

Gardens and play areas in pediatric settings are also believed to be beneficial in reducing stress and add to patient and staff satisfaction (Said, 2003; Said et al., 2005; Sherman et al., 2005; J. W. Varni et al., 2004). A post-occupancy evaluation was conducted at three healing gardens around a pediatric cancer center to determine whether the hospital garden was meeting the goals of reducing stress, restoring hope and energy and increasing consumer satisfaction. Results from behavioral observations, surveys and interviews showed that the garden with the most direct access was used the most. Further, emotional distress and perceived pain were lower for all garden users when in the garden as compared to when they were inside the building (Sherman et al., 2005).

Other studies conducted among adult patients in health care settings indicate that the built environment contributes significantly to overall satisfaction with the quality of care provided. A study conducted at a neurology outpatient waiting area before and after moving to a new location assessed how interior design changes in the new waiting areas affected environmental appraisals, self-reported stress and arousal, satisfaction ratings, and pulse readings. The results indicated that the new waiting area with interior design changes was associated with more positive environmental appraisals, improved mood, altered physiological state and greater reported satisfaction (Leather, Beale, Santos, Watts, & Lee, 2003). Interior design, architecture, housekeeping, privacy and the ambient environment were all perceived as sources of satisfaction by 380 discharged inpatients interviewed to determine relative contribution of environmental satisfaction to overall satisfaction (P. B. Harris, McBride, Ross, & Curtis, 2002). In another study conducted in three different settings – ambulatory care, acute care and long term care – eight consistent themes described what patients and family members look for in the health care built environment. In all three settings, they want an environment that facilitates a connection to staff and caregivers, is conducive to a sense of well-being and facilitates a connection to the outside world (Fowler et al., 1999).

Improving psychosocial outcomes — Summary and recommendations

Providing spaces for families in patient rooms enables parents, siblings and friends to visit and spend time with the patient and provides them the social interaction and support they need during this difficult time. Tools such as the Starlight Starbright programs, which help school-age children connect with a community of peers physically or online through the Internet, provide much needed social contact and intellectual stimulation. Studies show the therapeutic benefits of providing play spaces in health care settings that support play behavior and interaction among patients with different physical abilities and ages.

Adolescents have different social needs from younger children. Adolescent patients require a balance between privacy and intimacy and social interaction with people. Programmed amenities that provide distraction and remove the feeling of being in a hospital are likely to be preferred by adolescent patients.

Key recommendations:
- Incorporate age appropriate play areas
- Make minor modifications to improve ambience and attractiveness
- Incorporate single family patient rooms
- Provide space for families in patient rooms
- Incorporate accessible gardens
- Provide positive distractions such as artwork
- Provide education opportunities for children and adolescents
- Provide greater control over environment to patients and families

PROMOTING SAFETY THROUGH DESIGN

While promoting patient centered care is the foremost of the six aims for health care quality improvement set forth by the Institute of Medicine, quality of care cannot be achieved without drastic improvements in patient safety. Much of the literature on patient safety deals with adult settings. There are relatively fewer studies that deal with the impact of the physical environment on patient and staff safety in pediatric environments. Hence, findings from studies conducted in adult settings are described where they are likely relevant to pediatric environments as well.

Promoting Patient Safety

Pediatric patients are particularly susceptible to adverse outcomes in health care settings because they are often dependent upon an adult to communicate signs and symptoms to a health care provider. Children also differ epidemiologically from adult patients (Rice & Nelson, 2005). Children of different ages are exposed to different safety hazards. Loud noise, bright lights and choking hazards might pose risks to preterm infants. Older infants who can crawl might be at risk of falls and crib-related injuries as well as from choking on objects they put in their mouths. Exposure to airborne, waterborne and surface contact pathogens in the hospital environment poses a serious risk for nosocomial infections in pediatric patients, especially for those with weak immune systems. Facility layout and design may potentially influence medical errors and falls in pediatric environments, similar to adult acute care settings.

Reducing nosocomial infections

A strong body of research shows that the built environment influences the incidence of infection in hospitals and that, by careful consideration of environmental transmission routes – air, surface and water – in the design and operation of health care facilities, hospital-acquired infections can be reduced dramatically (Joseph, 2006b). Airborne infections are spread when dust and pathogens are released during hospital construction (Humphreys et al., 1991; Opal et al., 1986; Oren, Haddad, Finkelstein, & Rowe, 2001) due to contamination and malfunction of hospital ventilation systems (Kumari et al., 1998; Lutz, Jin, Rinaldi, Wickes, & Huycke, 2003; L. C. McDonald et al., 1998). Waterborne infections spread through direct contact (e.g., hydrotherapy), ingestion of contaminated water, indirect contact and inhalation of aerosols dispersed from water sources. The hands of health care staff are the principal cause of contact transmission from patient to patient (Chaberny, Schnitzler, Geiss, & Wendt, 2003; E. Larson, 1988; E. Larson, Albrecht, & O'Keefe, 2005). Several studies show that hand washing rates in many pediatric health care settings are extremely low – compliance rates in the range of 15 percent to 35 percent are typical (Cohen, Saiman, Cimiotti, & Larson, 2003; Hofer et al., 2007; E. Larson, Albrecht, & O'Keefe, 2005; R. S. Ulrich et al., 2004).

Nosocomial infection rates are higher in units that are understaffed, have a high patient census or bed occupancy rate or have high acuity patients. In a retrospective study, Archibald and colleagues (1997) linked the outbreak of Serratia marcescens in a pediatric cardiac intensive care unit to understaffing and overcrowding (high patient density). In a survey of 31 French pediatric wards, Jusot (2003) found that a lower incidence of hospital-acquired diarrhea was associated with restricting the mobility of the patient outside his or her room, keeping the patient's door closed and having fewer than 20 beds in the ward. Ben-Abraham and colleagues (2002) conducted a six-month comparative clinical study using retrospective data from 1992 (an open single space unit) and prospective surveillance from 1995 (individual rooms) to assess the effectiveness of the latter design on the control of nosocomial infections in critically ill pediatric patients. They found that the average number of nosocomial infections decreased significantly in the single room PICU unit. The length of stay was also significantly shorter in the single room PICU unit (25 +/- 6 in the open bay and 11 +/- 6 days in the single room). An in-depth literature study conducted in adult settings identified several studies showing that single rooms resulted in lower rates of nosocomial infection (R. S. Ulrich et al., 2004).

In addition to the factors commonly associated with nosocomial infection in adult settings, studies have identified other sources of infection unique to pediatric settings. For example, Avila-Aguero and colleagues (2004) obtained cultures from toys brought in by patients in a pediatric hospital and found that all the cultures tested positive for at least one infectious pathogen. After the toys were cleaned, bacterial growth decreased. An outbreak of P. aeruginosa in a pediatric oncology ward in Australia was linked to bath toys and a toy box containing water retaining toys (Buttery et al., 1999). Bubbles are commonly used in the process of therapeutic play, diversion and anxiety reduction in care delivery for young children. However, one study found that of a sample of 75 commercial bubble solutions (unopened and previously opened bottles), 50.6 percent had some microbial contaminant. Most solutions had a high count of bacteria (Dolan, Eberhart, & James, 2006). Another potential source of infection among patients is from pets used in pet therapy. Several studies have examined the health benefits of companionship from pets and the potential infection risks (Bouchard, Landry, Belles-Isles, & Gagnon, 2004; Brodie, Biley, & Shewring, 2002; Caprilli & Messeri, 2006). The studies suggest that benefits of pet therapy far outweigh risks provided proper hygiene precautions are taken for the animals, and staff and families are educated about associated safety issues (Brodie et al., 2002).

Literature reviews examining the impact of the physical environment on infections in health care settings found several studies indicating that improved air quality (through effective ventilation and filtration), design and maintenance of the heating, ventilation and air conditioning (HVAC) system, barrier precautions during construction and renovation activities, single bed rooms, visible and conveniently accessible hand washing sinks and alcohol-based gel dispensers, and regular cleaning and maintenance of water systems and point-of-use water fixtures are extremely effective in preventing nosocomial infections from airborne, waterborne and surface contact pathogens (Joseph, 2006b; R. S. Ulrich et al., 2004).

Ulrich and colleagues (2004) identified some low cost environmental approaches that might reduce nosocomial infections by increasing hand washing compliance. They identified several studies in which hospitals providing alcohol-based hand rubs in addition to sinks with soap and water increased the quality and frequency of hand washing. Further, providing alcohol-based hand-rub dispensers at the bedside was associated with increased hand washing compliance (R. S. Ulrich et al., 2004). Most of the studies described by Joseph (2006) and Ulrich and colleagues (2004) were conducted in health care settings housing adult populations. Immunocompromised patients were particularly susceptible to nosocomial infections

(Joseph, 2006b). Though fewer studies have been conducted among pediatric populations, it is likely that many infection control precautions and design features that can help prevent nosocomial infections in adult settings can be applied to pediatric settings as well.

Supporting communication between patients, families and staff

Health care practitioners are required to process different types of information and react quickly to the continuously changing conditions of their patients. Further, it is critical that practitioners – nurses, physicians, anesthetists and other clinical professionals – communicate vital patient information with each other to prevent replication of efforts, errors and other operational failures (McCarthy & Blumenthal, 2006; Uhlig, 2002; Uhlig, Brown, Nason, Camelio, & Kendall, 2002). Increased and open communication between patients, families and staff is an important element in promoting patient centered care.

Based on a conviction that better teamwork and communication are critical to improving patient safety, Dr. Paul Uhlig and colleagues started conducting multidisciplinary collaborative rounds at the patient bedside in 1999 in a cardiac surgery program in Concord, NH, (McCarthy & Blumenthal, 2006). This involved the entire care team (including the patient and family, bedside nurse, surgeon, nurse practitioner or physician assistant, social worker, spiritual care counselor, clinical and home care coordinators, a pharmacist, therapists, dietitian and rehabilitation specialists) participating in 10-minute briefings at the patient's bedside at the start of the day. The team reviews the patient's care plan, discusses medication and addresses anything that has gone wrong in the process in an open, blame-free environment (McCarthy & Blumenthal, 2006).

Following these changes, mortality rates declined, and both provider and patient satisfaction increased significantly (Uhlig, Brown, Nason, Camelio, & Kendall, 2002). Also, according to Uhlig, the rounds have become a way to reorient the care team to a "collaborative culture of interaction" (McCarthy & Blumenthal, 2006). Alton and colleagues (2006) also echo the benefits of integrating patients and families in bedside safety rounds initiated in a children's hospital. Families provided a critical perspective on the safety of the unit environment and were willing to partner with medical staff in promoting patient safety (Alton et al., 2006).

Becker (2007) suggests that for a culture of teamwork and communication to thrive, it may be important to provide the physical setting (as well as the technology infrastructure) that supports such behavior. For example, bedside rounds may not be feasible in small multi-occupancy rooms or on units without family waiting areas. A study at nine emergency departments to determine whether family centered care was supported by the staff revealed that some integration of family centered care principles was happening; the support was most consistent in the departments with programs that included the family. Of the nine emergency departments, lack of space in three department examination rooms limited families' participation in care (Eckle & MacLean, 2001). Environmental supports and visual cues likely to promote communication and interaction include:

- Different types of spaces for interactive team work
- Visual connections to facilitate information seeking and interaction
- Flexible workspaces
- Smaller unit size to foster interaction
- Neutral spaces that minimize professional and status hierarchies (Becker, 2007)

Reducing medical errors

More than 98,000 people die each year in U.S. hospitals due to medical errors (Kohn, Corrigan, & Donaldson, 1999). According to Reiling and colleagues (2004), while some errors (active failures) occur at the point of service (e.g., a nurse administering the wrong drug), most occur due to flaws in the health care system or facility design such as high noise levels or inadequate communication systems. Studies conducted in adult health care settings have linked inadequate light levels for visual tasks, frequent distractions and interruptions, and noisy and chaotic environments with medical errors (Buchanan, Barker, Gibson, Jiang, & Pearson, 1991; Flynn et al., 1999; Flynn et al., 1996; Tucker & Spear, 2006). Such environments add to the burden of stress experienced by staff and lead to errors.

Many new designs in adult hospitals are incorporating rooms that are all identical in configuration and orientation – same-handed patient rooms. That is, the patient is always on the same side of the room; gases and equipment are always located in the same position in every room. The premise for this design innovation is based on human factors research from other industries showing that increased standardization resulted in fewer errors by reducing the cognitive burden on the decision maker (Reiling et al., 2004). However, this innovation remains to be tested in health care.

While no studies examining the impact of environmental factors on medical errors have been conducted in pediatric settings, the findings from adult health care settings as they relate to noise, light and ergonomics may be relevant in pediatric settings as well. This is an important area for future research.

Reducing patient transfers

Patients are transferred from one room to another as often as three to six times during short stays in the hospital in order to receive the care that matches their level of acuity (Hendrich, Fay, & Sorrells, 2004; Hendrich & Lee, 2005). Patient transfers may often be accompanied by delays, misplaced medical records and lost information – all of which contribute to increased medical errors, loss of staff time and productivity (R. Ulrich & Zhu, 2007). If patients are misidentified, there can be serious implications for their health and safety. This is of particular concern for pediatric patients, especially infants, who may not be able to communicate critical information regarding identity and condition. A recent literature review by Ulrich and Zhu (2007) identified 22 scientific studies that examined the impact of transfers within the hospital on patient complications and the associated implications for designing safer, better hospitals. All studies except one (transport from a PICU) were conducted in adult settings, primarily dealing with transport from the ICU. According to the authors, there is a lack of rigorous research on the impact of design and building layout on transport-related complications (R. Ulrich & Zhu, 2007). However, certain design factors likely contribute to transport delays: restricted space and congestion and layouts that result in longer transport times. The studies suggest that elevator-dependent, vertical building layouts may negatively impact transport times and result in complications. The path-breaking study conducted by Hendrich and colleagues on the impact of acuity adaptable rooms on patient transfers in adult ICU settings provides strong justification for adopting acuity adaptable room and care models as a way to reduce patient transfers in adult settings (Hendrich et al., 2004; Hendrich & Lee, 2005).

Hendrich and colleagues (Hendrich et al., 2004; Hendrich & Lee, 2005) developed an innovative demonstration project called Cardiac Comprehensive Critical Care (CCCC) at Clarian Methodist Hospital in Indianapolis to address patient transfer and associated errors. The project provided different levels of care in a single patient room to minimize patient transfer as acuity levels changed. For this, each patient room was equipped with an acuity adaptable headwall, and all nurses on the unit were trained to respond to patients with varying acuity levels. The impact of this 56-bed variable acuity unit on different outcomes was measured by comparing two years of baseline data (before the move) and three years of data after the move. The project reports significant post-move improvement in many key areas: patient transfers decreased by 90 percent, medication errors by 70 percent. There was also a drastic reduction in the number of falls. This leading project demonstrated the potential impact of acuity adaptable care in dealing with patient flow and safety issues while improving the model of care. Many new projects across the country have adopted this model, though the impacts need to be assessed.

Reducing falls and injuries

Young children are susceptible to falls and injuries as they negotiate the physical environment. The unfamiliar environment of the hospital might pose additional hazards for institutionalized children. Falls from beds and cribs are the most common falls among children in hospitals (Warda, 2005). Historically, fall prevention strategies have not been a focus in pediatrics, and few studies focus on causes of falls or factors related to falls in pediatric settings (Buick, 2007). No known studies in pediatric settings examine the role of the physical environment as it relates to falls. Even in adult care settings, few studies examine the environmental correlates of falls. Bedrails that cause entrapment are potentially linked to falls in hospitalized adults as well as children (Hignett & Masud, 2006; Rice & Nelson, 2005).

Among specific interior design elements, flooring can contribute to incidence of falls (through slips) and the severity of injuries on impact (Drahota, Gal, & Windsor, 2007). Donald (2000) reports fewer falls of geriatric patients on vinyl floors as compared to carpeted floors in a rehabilitation ward. However, this study lacks sufficient power. Healy (1994), on the other hand, reports that adult patients suffer more injuries when they fall on vinyl floors versus carpeted floors. Simpson (2004) reports that the sub-floors may impact the injury from falls with the risk of fracture being lower for wooden sub-floors as compared to concrete sub-floors.

New hospital designs are incorporating decentralized nurse stations and alcoves with views into patient rooms with the premise that increased staff visibility will help reduce falls. In at least one prospective study, Hendrich and colleagues (2003) showed that falls among adult patients were reduced by two-thirds – from six-per-thousand patients to two-per-thousand – after a move from an old unit with centralized nursing station to a new unit with decentralized observation units. There is need for research to understand the effectiveness of this design intervention in pediatric settings. Patient rooms that include space for families support family presence – another factor which may potentially contribute to reduced falls among pediatric patients. However, no studies yet address this.

Promoting Staff Safety

While the focus of the safety movement in health care has been to prevent adverse outcomes among patients, health care staff is also exposed to occupational hazards that compromise staff safety and well-being. The work environment puts staff at risk for infection, injury and illness. In a recent literature review, Joseph (2007) examined the role of the physical environment in promoting health and safety among the health care team. The occupational hazards to which health care staff is exposed include airborne infections in the hospital as well as those acquired through direct contact with patients, back injuries from lifting and bending activities, loud noise, inadequate lighting, and poorly designed and crowded work stations. Night-shift staff often has poorly entrained circadian rhythms resulting in lack of sleep, stress and fatigue (Horowitz, Cade, Wolfe, & Czeisler, 2001a; Smith-Coggins, Rosekind, Buccino, Dinges, & Moser, 1997). These factors have direct implications for the health and safety of staff as well as the patients for whom staff is responsible. The majority of these studies were conducted with staff in adult care settings. However, it is very likely that most issues related to promoting staff safety are similar in both adult and pediatric settings.

Environmental design strategies such as improved air quality, filtration and provision of accessible hand washing sinks and alcohol-rub dispensers that result in reduced infections in patients are also likely to reduce risks of nosocomial infection among health care staff (Brady, 2005; Joseph, 2007).

Several studies show that exposure to intermittent bright light during the night shift is effective in adapting circadian rhythms of night-shift workers (Baehr, Fogg, & Eastman, 1999; Boivin & James, 2002; Crowley, Lee, Tseng, Fogg, & Eastman, 2003; Horowitz, Cade, Wolfe, & Czeisler, 2001b; Iwata, Ichii, & Egashira, 1997; Leppamaki, Partonen, Piiroinen, Haukka, & Lonnqvist, 2003). Exposure to bright light during the night shift may also improve mood and sleep (Leppamaki et al., 2003). In addition to bright-light exposure during the night, studies have shown that additional measures such as using dark sunglasses during the commute home and a regular early daytime sleep schedule ensure complete circadian adaptation to night-shift work (Boivin & James, 2002; Crowley et al., 2003; Horowitz et al., 2001b).

Ergonomic evaluations of the work area of different types of nursing staffs might provide solutions to problems specific to different groups. For example, based on an ergonomic evaluation of the work area of scrub nurses in the operating room, Gerbrands and colleagues (2004) provided short term solutions for reducing the neck and back problems experienced by this group as well as suggested guidelines for operating room design. Other interventions such as ceiling lifts have been very effective in reducing back injuries to staff in adult settings (Brophy, Achimore, & Moore-Dawson, 2001; A. Miller, Engst, Tate, & Yassi, 2006; Yassi et al., 2001). With growing obesity among children, it is plausible that ceiling lifts might be a more ergonomic solution to patient lifting in pediatric settings as well. There is a strong need for studies that evaluate the work environment of staff in pediatric settings to develop contextual ergonomics solutions.

Increasing Safety – Summary and Recommendations

Patient safety outcomes such as nosocomial infections and falls are directly impacted by environmental factors. Poor air quality, inadequate supports for hand washing and materials harboring infectious pathogens (e.g., toys) have all been linked with nosocomial infections in children. Research shows that single patient rooms are more effective than open bays in reducing the spread of nosocomial infection among pediatric patients, especially among immunocompromised patients. Environmental factors potentially contribute to falls in children though no studies have examined this in any detail. Other environmental hazards that may potentially lead to choking, tripping or burns among children should also be considered so that children's health care facilities are safer. The physical environment can also create conditions in which patient safety is compromised. For example, loud noises and inadequate meeting spaces are a barrier to communication and team work. Chaotic environments, poor ergonomics and low lighting levels may compound the burden of stress in staff and result in errors. New innovations such as acuity adaptable rooms appear promising in reducing patient transfers and associated adverse events; however, their applicability in pediatric settings needs to be tested. Studies in patient safety in pediatric settings have not yet focused on the role of the environment. This is an area where future research is needed.

Few studies have examined how the environment impacts staff safety in pediatric settings. Findings from adult settings that might be relevant in pediatric health care settings as well include reducing noise levels to reduce stress, improving task lighting for work surfaces, providing exposure to bright light to enable adaptation to circadian rhythms among night-shift workers and providing ergonomic solutions such as ceiling lifts to prevent injury among health care staff.

Key recommendations
- Install hand washing dispensers at the bedside
- Incorporate single family patient rooms
- Install HEPA filters in all areas housing immunocompromised patients
- Install ceiling lifts and adopt other ergonomic solutions

INCREASE STAFF EFFECTIVENESS IN PROVIDING CARE THROUGH DESIGN

According to a 2007 report released by PricewaterhouseCoopers Health Research Institute, the average nurse turnover rate in hospitals was 8.4 percent; the average voluntary turnover for first-year nurses was 27.1 percent. Additionally, one in seven hospitals reported a severe nurse vacancy rate of more than 20 percent (AHA, 2002). According to the Peter D. Hart Research Associates (2001) survey of registered nurses, the primary reason why nurses leave health care other than for retirement is to find a job that is less stressful and less physically demanding. To address the nursing shortage, one strategy proposed is to create healthy work environments. The physical environment of the health care workplace, along with other factors such as culture and work processes, impacts the health and safety of the health care workforce. Very few studies were found that specifically addressed the impact of the environment on staff effectiveness and health in pediatric settings. The majority of the studies described here were conducted among staff working in adult settings. However, it is likely that many of these findings are relevant in pediatric settings as well.

Decrease Staff Stress

Stress-related cortisol surges occur frequently in neonatal and pediatric critical care staff; and the majority of these surges are related to routine events such as coming to work, handing over to the next shift or presenting a patient during rounds (Fischer, Calame, Dettling, Zeier, & Fanconi, 2000). High levels of psychological stress have been associated with increased prevalence of nursing burnout. The tasks performed by the health care team involve a complex choreography of multiple activities including direct patient care, indirect care such as filling medications, coordination with care team members, accessing and communicating information, documentation of patient records and other housekeeping tasks (Lundgren & Segesten, 2001; Tucker & Spear, 2006).

Noise can be a source of stress for hospital staff and may interfere with their ability to work effectively (Topf, 1989). Noise-induced stress has been related to emotional exhaustion and burnout among critical care nurses (Topf & Dillon, 1988). In one study, health care staff perceived that the excessively high noise levels in the workplace interfered with their work and also impacted patient comfort and recovery (Bayo, Garcia, & Garcia, 1995). In a study on the impact of room acoustics, researchers found that during better acoustical conditions staff experienced fewer work demands and reported less pressure and strain (Blomkvist et al., 2005).

Laboratory studies of non-health care groups have found that noise often does not impair task performance when there is incentive to increase effort or pressure to maintain exacting standards. The laboratory findings suggest that adequate performance during noise is maintained by increasing effort, as evidenced by heightened cardiovascular response and other physiological mobilization (Parsons & Hartig, 2000). The research implies the possibility that health care staff may be able to maintain performance during some noisy situations, but at the cost of exerting greater effort and becoming more fatigued. Staff reactions to noise include irritability, anxiety, impaired judgment, altered perceptions and difficulty concentrating (Bailey & Timmons, 2005). A study on noise in a PICU revealed that staff conversation was responsible for most noise while medical equipment, patient interventions, telephones, alarm and mechanical systems were also responsible in causing high levels of noise (Morrison, Haas, Shaffner, Garrett, & Fackler, 2003). Recommendations for architectural designs to reduce noise included using sound insulating material for floors, walls and ceilings (R. J. Berens & Weigle, 1996; Blomkvist et al., 2005).

Providing access to nature through gardens in hospital settings has been shown to increase staff satisfaction as well as foster access to social support, positive escape and recuperation from stressful clinical situations (Cooper-Marcus & Barnes, 1999). Healing gardens in hospitals can provide a setting for staff to conduct various therapies with patients, for staff to retreat from the stressors within the walls of the hospital and provide an opportunity for patient-visitor interaction (Cooper-Marcus & Barnes, 1999). Positive mood change and reduced stress was reported within post-occupancy studies of patients and families who use hospital gardens (Said et al., 2005; Sherman et al., 2005; Whitehouse et al., 2001). Key design considerations for optimal garden use in hospitals include: visibility, accessibility, familiarity, quiet sound environment, comfort and unambiguously positive art (Cooper-Marcus & Barnes, 1999). In an exploratory study conducted at a children's hospital, researchers found that an outside view through a window along with the type of view was related to acute stress and alertness among nurses (Pati & Barach, In Review). In a pediatric cancer center, staff used gardens to walk through or to sit and eat in, but rarely interacted with features intended for active engagement. The data suggested that emotional distress and pain are lower for all when in the gardens than when inside the hospital (Sherman et al., 2005).

Increase Staff Satisfaction

An ongoing struggle for staff in pediatric settings is to balance parent satisfaction with the care provided and job satisfaction among nurses (Goldschmidt & Gordin, 2006). Staff concerns are teamwork, communication and continuity of nursing care. Nurses have expressed concerns about providing care in single room NICUs; nurses said that providing sufficient staff coverage was difficult due to decreased patient visibility and greater distances between patients. Larger units also present unique communication, staff education and quality improvement challenges (W. F. Walsh, McCullough, & White, 2006).

A human factors evaluation compared perceptions and performance of the neonatal intensive care staff when moving from an open bay to a private room model (Schoenbeck, 2006). Staff perceived that the private room model improved the quality of the physical environmental conditions, interaction with the families of the infant and overall patient care. However, they felt that the interaction among team members worsened when working in the private room model (Schoenbeck, 2006). Another study compared staff members' perceptions of their working environments across three different types of NICU settings (all single family rooms, single family and open bay, all open bay). The researchers found that staff members in the all single family room NICU unit were the most satisfied (D. D. Harris et al., 2006). There is an increasing trend towards single family rooms in the NICU and future studies should focus on the impact of these designs on patients and families as well as staff.

A study examining the change in staff satisfaction on the opening of a dedicated pediatric emergency department reported an increased level of confidence and satisfaction with regard to the new physical environment (Judkins, 2003). The change in the physical environment (renovations, new construction) in which care is provided appears to enhance the level of staff satisfaction (D. D. Harris et al., 2006; Judkins, 2003). Incorporating elements of a healing environment (e.g., views of nature, natural light, soothing colors, therapeutic sounds and the interaction of family members) optimizes staff satisfaction, morale and retention (Altimier, 2004).

In a post-occupancy evaluation of a children's hospital, staff was surveyed on the physical environment of the existing facility; the results indicated the staff was not satisfied with the existing facility due to lack of space, inadequate number of private areas, the location of nursing station and the amount of natural lighting. The post-occupancy evaluation results contributed to specific changes to the built environment, which included larger bathrooms with showers, larger closet/storage space, larger activity spaces, staff break room, a dining room, wheelchair storage in each child's bedroom and a large outdoor recreation area. Additionally, this study revealed that higher staff satisfaction with the built environment structure and aesthetics was associated with higher coworker relationship satisfaction (J. W. Varni et al., 2004).

Increase Staff Effectiveness and Efficiency

It is becoming increasingly clear that poorly designed physical environments along with other factors such as lack of social support and an unsupportive work culture, reduce the effectiveness of staff in providing care and potentially lead to medical errors. The design of the layout of the nursing unit, providing ample lighting capabilities, ergonomic sensitivities and sound control can improve staff effectiveness and efficiency. However, this is an area where there is relatively less research, especially in pediatric settings.

Nurses spend approximately one-third of their time walking on the unit between patient rooms, nurses station and supply areas, which, in turn, results in fatigue (Burgio, Engel, Hawkins, McCorick, & Scheve, 1990). Bringing staff and supplies closer to patients may potentially reduce time spent walking and increase time spent in direct patient care activities. Several studies revealed that, due to the unit layout, time saved walking was translated into more time spent on patient-care activities and the interaction with family members (Shepley, 2002; Shepley & Davies, 2003; Sturdavant, 1960; Trites, Galbraith, Sturdavant, & Leckwart, 1970). Further, nurses spent a lot of time finding people, equipment and supplies and are often interrupted while working. In one study, a hospital nurse was interrupted 43 times during a 10-hour period, including 10 instances when necessary materials, equipment and personnel were unavailable (Potter et al., 2004).

Inadequate lighting coupled with a chaotic health care environment is likely to lead to errors. Very few studies have focused specifically on the impact of different types of lighting conditions on staff work performance in hospitals. One study examined the effect of different illumination levels on pharmacists' prescription-dispensing error rates. It found that error rates were reduced when work-surface light levels were relatively high (Buchanan et al., 1991). In this study, three different illumination levels were evaluated (450 lux; 1,100 lux; and 1,500 lux). Medication-dispensing error rates were significantly lower (2.6 percent) at an illumination level of 1,500 lux (highest level) compared to an error rate of 3.8 percent at 450 lux. This is consistent with findings from office settings that show that task performance improves with increased light levels (Boyce, Hunter, & Howlett, 2003). Additional research is needed to assess the impact that lighting may have in reducing errors and increasing efficiency in the patient room and staff work areas.

Increasing Staff Effectiveness — Summary and Recommendations

Satisfied and effective personnel are integral components to providing quality care in pediatric hospitals, though few studies have focused specifically on staff outcomes in children's health care environments. However, findings from studies conducted among staff in adult settings likely apply to pediatric settings as well. Excessive noise is a stressor for staff and leads to fatigue and burnout. In contrast, exposure to gardens is a source of satisfaction, improved mood and reduced stress. Some studies have examined the impact of unit design and interior design changes on staff satisfaction. They suggest that staff prefer and have less stress in single family rooms in the NICU. However, in some cases, staff members in NICUs have expressed concerns over single patient room designs, believing that they make it more difficult for them to monitor and effectively care for their patients. Unit renovations and physical design improvements are associated with greater staff satisfaction. Some studies conducted in adult settings suggest that unit layouts designed to reduce walking, to increase staff access to patients, and to place equipment and supplies closer to staff result in increased efficiency. However, further research is needed in pediatric settings.

Key recommendations
- Increase visual access and accessibility to patients
- Incorporate accessible gardens
- Improve ambience and attractiveness

CONCLUSIONS AND FUTURE RESEARCH DIRECTIONS

A growing body of research shows that the physical design of health care settings contributes to the negative outcomes such as stress, falls, nosocomial infections and errors experienced so frequently in health care. On the other hand, thoughtful evidence-based facility design can help bring the patient, staff and families into the center of the health care experience, increase patient safety in the health care environment and advance the overall quality of care provided. *Evidence for Innovation* clearly demonstrates that the physical environment of pediatric settings impacts clinical, developmental, psychosocial and safety outcomes among patients and families. The physical environment is a key component of providing patient and family centered care and increasing safety and overall quality of care in pediatric settings.

The studies described in this literature review cover a range of different pediatric populations, preterm infants, toddlers, young children and adolescents, as well as staff and families. Within children's environments, a majority of the studies focus on NICU settings as compared to general pediatric settings. Design innovations such as incorporating single family rooms and decentralizing nurses stations to improve quality of care appear to be gaining acceptance in NICU settings. It is not clear from the literature whether such innovations are being incorporated in general pediatric settings as well. More studies focus on inpatient settings as compared to ambulatory care settings or long-term care settings for children.

The number of studies that deal with issues specific to pediatric settings is relatively small compared to those in adult settings. Especially, there are few studies on the impact of facility design on staff and families in pediatric settings. In areas such as these, we have extrapolated from studies conducted in adult settings. However, we need to understand the design dynamics of providing care in pediatric settings specifically and how that impacts staff health, safety and effectiveness.

Many studies focusing on children tend to elicit opinions and perceptions from families and staff as a proxy for patient perceptions. There is great merit in obtaining first hand information from sick children about their hospital experiences and their interaction with the care environment. A majority of rigorous experimental and quasi experimental studies has been conducted in NICU settings. More rigorous research is needed in general pediatric settings on a range of topics. Many studies have not been replicated. To generate stronger, consistent recommendations, we need replication on several topics.

While existing research is promising, several gaps exist in the literature. In some cases, topics have been explored in adult settings though not in pediatric settings (indicated below as "A"). In other cases, there is a complete lack of information, and research is needed (indicated below as "N"). Listed below are questions that need to be addressed through future research in pediatric facilities. The list is not exhaustive, but is meant to give some direction for future research.

TABLE 3

Opportunities for Future Study
A = Studies in adults, not in pediatrics   N = Needs study

Noise related studies

- How does noise affect sleep, delirium and coping among children in pediatric settings? (A)
- How do noise levels affect family members' anxiety in pediatric settings? (N)
- Is some noise good; what threshold of noise levels do children find disturbing? What appropriate acoustical conditions strike the balance between sensory stimulation and disturbance? (N)
- What environmental interventions are used to reduce noise levels in different pediatric settings? (A)

Impact of light

- Is exposure to natural light among children and adolescents effective in reducing depression and improving outcomes such as reduced perception of pain and intake of pain medication? (A)
- How does exposure to natural light during the work day impact staff stress and satisfaction? (N)

Impact of positive distractions

- How do window views affect outcomes among pediatric patients? (A)
- Does the content of artwork (i.e., nature vs. abstract image) impact stress and anxiety among pediatric patients? (A)

Impact of unit and room design

- How do decentralized nursing stations impact staff effectiveness in providing care? (N)
- Should some rooms in pediatric facilities have the option of multiple occupancy to allow for socialization and siblings? (N)
- Do decentralized nurses stations and family space in patient rooms help to reduce patient injuries in pediatric hospitals? (N)
- Will providing family space in patient rooms and allowing family presence on the unit help reduce patient and family stress and anxiety and increase participation in care and ease in transitioning to home setting? (N)
- Will single patient rooms increase family presence on the unit and participation in care? (N)

Impact of design on errors

- Can patient transfers and related errors be reduced by designing acuity adaptable patient rooms? (A)
- How do noise, lighting and workspace design impact medical errors in pediatric settings? (A)

TRANSFORMING CARE IN CHILDREN'S HOSPITALS THROUGH ENVIRONMENTAL DESIGN APPENDIX

The appendix has the following components:

1. Design concepts (Table A): Review of the existing research led to design concepts, which were then examined according to measured outcome variables and number of studies cited within the literature review.

2. Article analysis methodology (Table B): Articles were assessed individually for quality, rigor and relevance to the study at hand. The methodology used to analyze individual articles is described.

3. Article analysis (Table C): A sample of the studies (77 studies) was analyzed in detail utilizing a criteria checklist.

Design Concepts

When reviewing the existing evidence on the impact of the physical environment on pediatric health care facilities, design concepts and/or strategies were found within each study examined. These concepts can be found within the body of knowledge of the literature review as well as in Table A, which explores the relationship between the design concepts and the associated patient, family or staff outcome. The number of studies that measure the same relationship (between design concept and outcome) and whether the outcome has a positive or negative impact is noted.

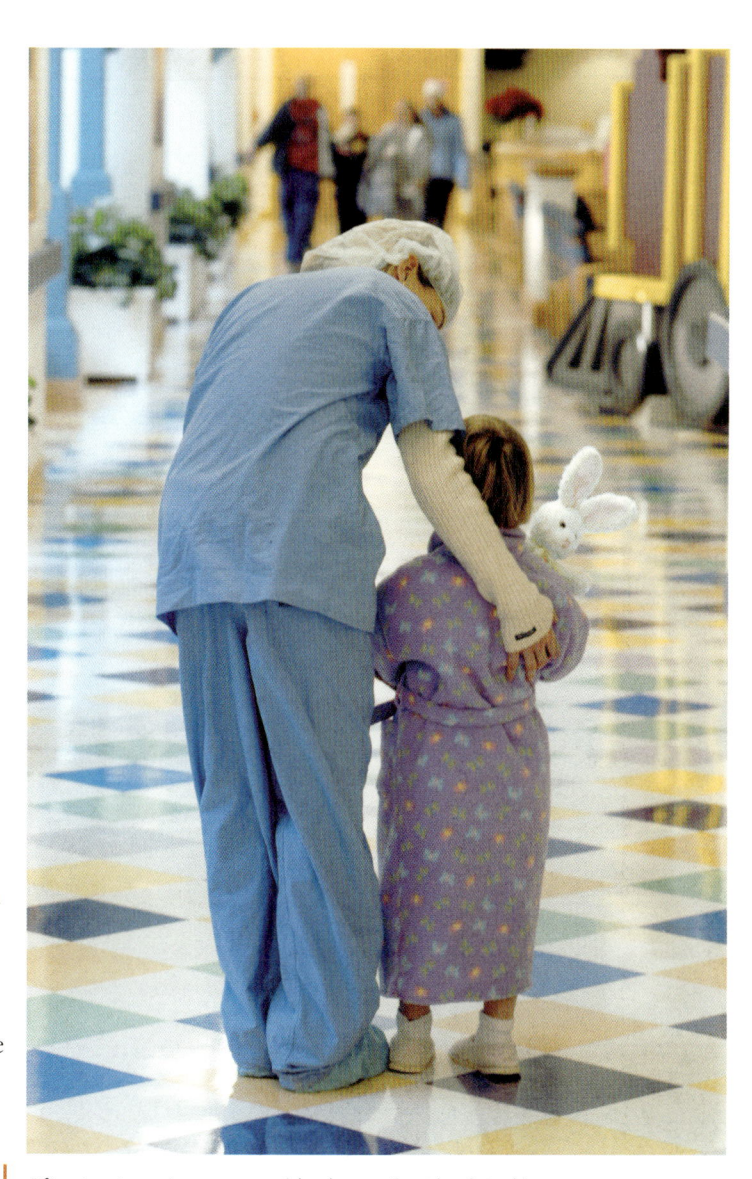

After treatment, a nurse guides her patient back to his room. Photo by Cynthia Brodoway, Alfred I. duPont Hospital for Children, Wilmington, DE

APPENDIX | TABLE A: DESIGN CONCEPTS AND ASSOCIATED OUTCOMES

CHILDREN IN HEALTH CARE ENVIRONMENTS

Literature Review Contents	Design Concept Found Within Section of Literature Review	Staff Outcome	Family Outcome	Patient Outcome	Negative Impact	Positive Impact	# of Studies	References Cited
Advancing patient centered and family centered care through design	Design environments to involve family in child's care		Improved satisfaction with care			x	5	Henriksen et al. 2007; Saunders et al. 2003; Macnab, Thiessen and Hinto 2000; Forsythe 1998; Meyer et. al. 1994
			Decreased parental stress			x	5	Henriksen et al. 2007; Saunders et al. 2003; Macnab, Thiessen and Hinto 2000; Forsythe 1998; Meyer et. al. 1994
			Increased parental comfort			x	5	Henriksen et al. 2007; Saunders et al. 2003; Macnab, Thiessen and Hinto 2000; Forsythe 1998; Meyer et. al. 1994
			Increased parental competence with post discharge care			x	5	Henriksen et al. 2007; Saunders et al. 2003; Macnab, Thiessen and Hinto 2000; Forsythe 1998; Meyer et. al. 1994
			Improved success with breastfeeding			x	5	Henriksen et al. 2007; Saunders et al. 2003; Macnab, Thiessen and Hinto 2000; Forsythe 1998; Meyer et. al. 1994
				Shortened hospital lengths of stay		x	5	Henriksen et al. 2007; Saunders et al. 2003; Macnab, Thiessen and Hinto 2000; Forsythe 1998; Meyer et. al. 1994
				Decreased readmissions post discharge		x	5	Henriksen et al. 2007; Saunders et al. 2003; Macnab, Thiessen and Hinto 2000; Forsythe 1998; Meyer et. al. 1994
		Increased staff satisfaction				x	5	Henriksen et al. 2007; Saunders et al. 2003; Macnab, Thiessen and Hinto 2000; Forsythe 1998; Meyer et. al. 1994
	Design environments with patients and families as the core focus			Improved clinical and physiological outcomes		x		Henriksen et al. 2007; Saunders et al. 2003; Macnab, Thiessen and Hinto 2000; Forsythe 1998; Meyer et. al. 1994
	Design environment to provide greater control	Supported psychological outcomes	Supported psychological outcomes	Supported psychological outcomes		x		Henriksen et al. 2007; Saunders et al. 2003; Macnab, Thiessen and Hinto 2000; Forsythe 1998; Meyer et. al. 1994
	Design environment to protect confidentiality and privacy	Supported psychological outcomes	Supported psychological outcomes	Supported psychological outcomes		x		Henriksen et al. 2007; Saunders et al. 2003; Macnab, Thiessen and Hinto 2000; Forsythe 1998; Meyer et. al. 1994
	Design environment to facilitate communication and participation in care	Supported psycho-logical outcomes	Suporedt psychological outcomes	Supported psychological outcomes		x		Henriksen et al. 2007; Saunders et al. 2003; Macnab, Thiessen and Hinto 2000; Forsythe 1998; Meyer et. al. 1994

APPENDIX | TABLE A: DESIGN CONCEPTS AND ASSOCIATED OUTCOMES | 49

Literature Review Contents	Design Concept Found Within Section of Literature Review	Staff Outcome	Family Outcome	Patient Outcome	Negative Impact	Positive Impact	# of Studies	References Cited
Improving Clinical and Physiological Outcomes								
Impact of noise on sleep and developmental outcomes	Design closed bay environments	Reduced noise	Reduced noise	Reduced noise		x	2	Couper et al. 2004; Berens 1999
	Design single occupancy rooms with closed doors			Reduced noise levels at patient bedside		x	1	Ulrich et al. 2004
	Utilize high performance sound absorbing acoustical ceiling tiles	Reduced noise and reverberation	Reduced noise and reverberation	Reduced noise and reverberation		x	1	Blomkvist et. al 2005
	Eliminate excessive noise levels in NICU			Reduced stress		x	3	Gray and Philbin 2005; Bremmer, Byers and Kiehl 2003
				Decreased detrimental development effects		x	3	Gray and Philbin 2005; Bremmer, Byers and Kiehl 2003
				Reinforced auditory system development & attention		x	3	Gray and Philbin 2005; Bremmer, Byers and Kiehl 2003
	Alter noise levels within infant incubator (place earmuffs on the infants, cover incubator, install sound absorbing panel in incubator, put sound absorbing foam next to infant)			Demonstrated physiological benefits for infant development and convalescence		x	5	Johnson 2001; Saunders 1995; Bellieni et al. 2003; Zahr and Traversay 1995; Walsh et al. 2005
				Decreased heart rate		x	2	Johnson 2001; Zahr and Traversay 1995
				Decreased respiratory rate		x	2	Johnson 2001; Zahr and Traversay 1995
				Increased sleep state and sleep/awake changes		x	2	Johnson 2001; Zahr and Traversay 1995
				Increased oxygen saturation		x	2	Johnson 2001; Zahr and Traversay 1995
	Install weather stripping	Reduced noise	Reduced noise	Reduced noise		x	1	Walsh et al. 2005
	Replace metal trash cans with rubber ones	Reduced noise	Reduced noise	Reduced noise		x	1	Walsh et al. 2005
	Install carpet	Reduced noise	Reduced noise	Reduced noise		x	1	Walsh et al. 2005

APPENDIX | TABLE A: DESIGN CONCEPTS AND ASSOCIATED OUTCOMES

Literature Review Contents	Design Concept Found Within Section of Literature Review	Staff Outcome	Family Outcome	Patient Outcome	Negative Impact	Positive Impact	# of Studies	References Cited
Impact of noise on sleep and developmental outcomes	Install sound-absorbing materials (floors, walls, and/or ceilings)	Reduced noise	Reduced noise	Reduced noise		x	3	Walsh et al. 2005; Ulrich et. al 2004; Blomkist et al. 2005
	Use privacy curtains	Reduced noise	Reduced noise	Reduced noise		x	1	Byers, Waugh and Lowman 2006
	Install noise indicator lights near nurses work stations	Reduced noise	Reduced noise	Reduced noise		x	1	Thear and Wittmann-Price 2006
	Structurally reduce noise admitted by doors	Reduced noise	Reduced noise	Reduced noise		x	1	Thear and Wittmann-Price 2006
	Make equipment alterations and changes to reduce the noise environment	Reduced noise	Reduced noise	Reduced noise		x	1	Byers, Waugh and Lowman 2006
Impact of lighting on developmental outcomes	Maximize exposure to light for neonates			Lowered serum bilirubin		x	2	Giunta and Rath 1969; McColl and Veitch 2001
				Retinal damage	x		2	Ackerman, Sherwonit and Fisk 1989; Mann et al. 1986
	Provide cycled lighting in NICUs			Improved sleep		x	4	Miller et al. 1995; Brandon, Holditch-Davis and Belyea 2002; Mann et. al. 1986; Blackburn and Patterson 1991
				Improved weight gain		x	4	Miller et al. 1995; Brandon, Holditch-Davis and Belyea 2002; Mann et. al. 1986; Blackburn and Patterson 1991
				Enhanced motor coordination		x	1	Miller et al. 1995
				Reduced days on ventilator		x	1	Miller et al. 1995
				Increased oral feeding		x	1	Miller et al. 1995
	Reduce ambient lighting conditions in nurseries			Improved retinopathy outcomes		x	2	Ackerman, Sherwonit and Fisk 1989; Mann et al. 1986
	Maximize exposure to light for adults (possible link to older hospitalized children)			Reduced depression		x	3	Beauchemin and Hays 1996; Benedetti et al. 2001; Walch et al. 2005

APPENDIX | TABLE A: DESIGN CONCEPTS AND ASSOCIATED OUTCOMES | 51

Literature Review Contents	Design Concept Found Within Section of Literature Review	Staff Outcome	Family Outcome	Patient Outcome	Negative Impact	Positive Impact	# of Studies	References Cited
Impact of lighting on developmental outcomes	Maximize exposure to light for adults (possible link to older hospitalized children)			Reduced intake of pain medication		x	3	Beauchemin and Hays 1996; Benedetti et al. 2001; Walch et al. 2005
				Reduced length of stay		x	3	Beauchemin and Hays 1996; Benedetti et al. 2001; Walch et al. 2005
Impact of the environment on stress	Use music as background noise		Increased comfort level	Increased comfort level		x	2	Polkki, Vehvilainen and Pietla 2001; Brice and Barclay 2007
			Decreased anxiety	Decreased anxiety		x	2	Polkki, Vehvilainen and Pietla 2001; Brice and Barclay 2007
	Play recorded lullabies during immunizations			Reduced overall distress		x	2	Malone 1996; Megel, Houser and Gleaves 1998
	Spend time in a garden			Increased independence		x	2	Said and Abu Bakar 2004; Said 2003
				Reduced emotional disturbance		x	3	Said and Abu Bakar 2004; Said 2003; Sherman et al. 2005
				Increased cheerful and agile behaviors		x	3	Said and Abu Bakar 2004; Said 2003; Sherman et al. 2005
				Increased cooperative and obedient behavior		x	2	Said and Abu Bakar 2004; Said 2003
				Reduced overall distress		x	3	Said and Abu Bakar 2004; Said 2003; Sherman et al. 2005
				Increased feelings of wellness		x	2	Said and Abu Bakar 2004; Said 2003
	Utilize music within the NICU			Increased oxygen saturation		x	2	Arnon et al. 2006; Shepley 2006
				Decreased heart rate		x	2	Arnon et al. 2006; Shepley 2006
				Decreased behavioral issues		x	2	Arnon et al. 2006; Shepley 2006

APPENDIX | TABLE A: DESIGN CONCEPTS AND ASSOCIATED OUTCOMES

Literature Review Contents	Design Concept Found Within Section of Literature Review	Staff Outcome	Family Outcome	Patient Outcome	Negative Impact	Positive Impact	# of Studies	References Cited
Impact of the environment on stress	Utilize music within the NICU			Decreased incidence of respiratory pause		x	2	Arnon et al. 2006; Shepley 2006
	Utilize live music during music therapy with infants			Decreased heart rate		x	1	Arnon et al. 2006
				Decreased sleep/awake state		x	1	Arnon et al. 2006
Impact of the environment on perception of pain and medication use	Utilize music therapy			Decreased use of sedatives during procedures		x	2	Walworth 2005; Loewy et al. 2005
				Effective method for induced sleep		x	2	Walworth 2005; Loewy et al. 2005
				Decreased pain perception		x	1	Malone 1996
				Decreased observable distress		x	1	Malone 1996
	Utilize music before and after invasive procedures			Decreased pain perception		x	2	Malone 1996; Wolitzky et al. 2005
	Utilize virtual reality games and programs during painful procedures			Decreased anxiety		x	2	Malone 1996; Wolitzky et al. 2005
				Increased narrative detail remembered from procedure		x	2	Malone 1996; Wolitzky et al. 2005

Improving psychosocial outcomes

Literature Review Contents	Design Concept Found Within Section of Literature Review	Staff Outcome	Family Outcome	Patient Outcome	Negative Impact	Positive Impact	# of Studies	References Cited
Improve coping skills	Provide ample family space in patient rooms			Aided in distraction	x	x	5	Davidson et al. 2007; Bers, Gonzalez-Heydrich and DeMaso 2003; Junior, Coutinho and Ferreira 2006; Robb 2000; Boyd and Hunsberger 1998
				Increased verbal and emotional expression		x	5	Davidson et al. 2007; Bers, Gonzalez-Heydrich and DeMaso 2003; Junior, Coutinho and Ferreira 2006; Robb 2000; Boyd and Hunsberger 1998
				Increased familiarity		x	5	Davidson et al. 2007; Bers, Gonzalez-Heydrich and DeMaso 2003; Junior, Coutinho and Ferreira 2006; Robb 2000; Boyd and Hunsberger 1998
				Promoted independent activities		x	5	Davidson et al. 2007; Bers, Gonzalez-Heydrich and DeMaso 2003; Junior, Coutinho and Ferreira 2006; Robb 2000; Boyd and Hunsberger 1998

APPENDIX | TABLE A: DESIGN CONCEPTS AND ASSOCIATED OUTCOMES | 53

Literature Review Contents	Design Concept Found Within Section of Literature Review	Staff Outcome	Family Outcome	Patient Outcome	Negative Impact	Positive Impact	# of Studies	References Cited
Improve coping skills	Utilize a kaleidoscope during needle-stick procedures			Decreased pain perception		x	1	Vessey, Carlson and McGill 1994
				Reduced behavioral distress		x	1	Vessey, Carlson and McGill 1994
	Utilize virtual reality games and programs during painful procedures			Reduced pain		x	2	Gershon et al. 2003; Wolitzky et al. 2005
				Reduced anxiety ratings		x	2	Gershon et al. 2003; Wolitzky et al. 2005
				Reduced pulse		x	2	Gershon et al. 2003; Wolitzky et al. 2005
				Reduced behavioral issues		x	2	Gershon et al. 2003; Wolitzky et al. 2005
	Design quiet rooms with ambience (attractiveness) which could include: colored paint on walls, carpeted floors and artwork within space			Reduced aggression ratings		x	1	Glod et al. 1994
				Increased calming interventions		x	1	Glod et al. 1994
Provide social support: Peer to peer communication	Maximize contact with peers of pediatric and adolescent patients			Increased social and communication skills		x	3	Said and Abu Bakar 2004; Said et al. 2005; Fels et al. 2001
				Aided in development of self-confidence and independence		x	3	Said and Abu Bakar 2004; Said et al. 2005; Fels et al. 2001
	Utilize interactive online virtual communities			Reduced pain		x	6	Battles and Wiener 2002; Brokstein, Cohen and Walco 2002; Holden et al. 1999; Rode et al. 1998; Bush, Huchital and Simonian 2002
				Reduced distress		x	6	Battles and Wiener 2002; Brokstein, Cohen and Walco 2002; Holden et al. 1999; Rode et al. 1998; Bush, Huchital and Simonian 2002
				Reduced fear with hospitalization, disease/illness		x	6	Battles and Wiener 2002; Brokstein, Cohen and Walco 2002; Holden et al. 1999; Rode et al. 1998; Bush, Huchital and Simonian 2002
				Minimized isolation		x	6	Battles and Wiener 2002; Brokstein, Cohen and Walco 2002; Holden et al. 1999; Rode et al. 1998; Bush, Huchital and Simonian 2002

APPENDIX | TABLE A: DESIGN CONCEPTS AND ASSOCIATED OUTCOMES

Literature Review Contents	Design Concept Found Within Section of Literature Review	Staff Outcome	Family Outcome	Patient Outcome	Negative Impact	Positive Impact	# of Studies	References Cited
Provide social support: Peer to peer communication	Utilize interactive online virtual communities (example, Starbright World)			Increased willingness to return for treatment		x	6	Battles and Wiener 2002; Brokstein, Cohen and Walco 2002; Holden et al. 1999; Rode et al. 1998; Holden et al. 2001; Bush, Huchital and Simonian 2002
				Increased sense of peer support		x	6	Battles and Wiener 2002; Brokstein, Cohen and Walco 2002; Holden et al. 1999; Rode et al. 1998; Holden et al. 2001; Bush, Huchital and Simonian 2002
				Increased knowledge on disease/illness		x	6	Battles and Wiener 2002; Brokstein, Cohen and Walco 2002; Holden et al. 1999; Rode et al. 1998; Holden et al. 2001; Bush, Huchital and Simonian 2002
				Increased responsibility for managing disease/illness		x	6	Battles and Wiener 2002; Brokstein, Cohen and Walco 2002; Holden et al. 1999; Rode et al. 1998; Holden et al. 2001; Bush, Huchital and Simonian 2002
				Increased ability to cope with disease/illness		x	6	Battles and Wiener 2002; Brokstein, Cohen and Walco 2002; Holden et al. 1999; Rode et al. 1998; Holden et al. 2001; Bush, Huchital and Simonian 2002
				Increased energetic mood		x	6	Battles and Wiener 2002; Brokstein, Cohen and Walco 2002; Holden et al. 1999; Rode et al. 1998; Holden et al. 2001; Bush, Huchital and Simonian 2002
				Decreased feelings of depression		x	6	Battles and Wiener 2002; Brokstein, Cohen and Walco 2002; Holden et al. 1999; Rode et al. 1998; Holden et al. 2001; Bush, Huchital and Simonian 2002
	Employ videoconferencing capabilities with robotics			Promoted engagement and interaction with peers and classroom		x	4	Fels et al. 2001; Battles and Wiener 2002; Rassin, Gutman and Silner 2004; Bers et al. 2001
				Increased positive contributions and ideas to remote discussion		x	4	Fels et al. 2001; Battles and Wiener 2002; Rassin, Gutman and Silner 2004; Bers et al. 2001
Encourage opportunities for play and education	Utilize the activity of play as a therapeutic tool with pediatric patients			Reduced tension		x	11	Junior, Coutinho and Ferreira 2006; Carvalho and Begnis 2006; Haiat, Bar-Mor and Shochat 2003; Gariepy and Howe 2003; Craddock 2003; Naka et al. 2002; Urazoe et al. 2001; Pass and Bolig 1993; Wishon and Brown 1991; Vessey and Mahon 1990; Ispa, Barrett and Yanghee 1988

APPENDIX | TABLE A: DESIGN CONCEPTS AND ASSOCIATED OUTCOMES | 55

Literature Review Contents	Design Concept Found Within Section of Literature Review	Staff Outcome	Family Outcome	Patient Outcome	Negative Impact	Positive Impact	# of Studies	References Cited
Encourage opportunities for play and education	Utilize the activity of play as a therapeutic tool with pediatric patients			Reduced anxiety		x	11	Junior, Coutinho and Ferreira 2006; Carvalho and Begnis 2006; Haiat, Bar-Mor and Shochat 2003; Gariepy and Howe 2003; Craddock 2003; Naka et al. 2002; Urazoe et al. 2001; Pass and Bolig 1993; Wishon and Brown 1991; Vessey and Mahon 1990; Ispa, Barrett and Yanghee 1988
				Reduced anger and conflict		x	11	Junior, Coutinho and Ferreira 2006; Carvalho and Begnis 2006; Haiat, Bar-Mor and Shochat 2003; Gariepy and Howe 2003; Craddock 2003; Naka et al. 2002; Urazoe et al. 2001; Pass and Bolig 1993; Wishon and Brown 1991; Vessey and Mahon 1990; Ispa, Barrett and Yanghee 1988
				Reduced frustration		x	11	Junior, Coutinho and Ferreira 2006; Carvalho and Begnis 2006; Haiat, Bar-Mor and Shochat 2003; Gariepy and Howe 2003; Craddock 2003; Naka et al. 2002; Urazoe et al. 2001; Pass and Bolig 1993; Wishon and Brown 1991; Vessey and Mahon 1990; Ispa, Barrett and Yanghee 1988
	Expose children to medical equipment before procedures			Reduced anxiety		x	1	Ispa, Barrett and Yanghee 1988
	Control unnecessary sources of stimulation in play areas (such as create a neutral background)			Increased time spent in play behaviors		x	1	Eisert, Kulka and Moore 1988
	Decrease clutter in play areas			Increased accessibility		x	1	Eisert, Kulka and Moore 1988
	Improve storage in play areas			Encouraged exploration and self-initiation		x	1	Eisert, Kulka and Moore 1988
	Use color and variety to define space in play areas			Encouraged exploration and self-initiation		x	1	Eisert, Kulka and Moore 1988
	Display toys to increase accessibility			Increased time spent in play behaviors		x	1	Eisert, Kulka and Moore 1988

APPENDIX | TABLE A: DESIGN CONCEPTS AND ASSOCIATED OUTCOMES

Literature Review Contents	Design Concept Found Within Section of Literature Review	Staff Outcome	Family Outcome	Patient Outcome	Negative Impact	Positive Impact	# of Studies	References Cited
Encourage opportunities for play and education	Display toys in play areas for differing individuals (age, physical and mental abilities)			Increased time spent in play behaviors		x	1	Eisert, Kulka and Moore 1988
				Increased ability for play behavior		x	1	Eisert, Kulka and Moore 1988
	Design a structured playroom setting			Increased conversation engagements		x	3	Pass and Bolig 1993; Vavili 2000; Clatworthy 1981
				Increased play behaviors (feeding the fish)		x	3	Pass and Bolig 1993; Vavili 2000; Clatworthy 1981
	Incorporate technology (video games) to serve as an educational tool			Increased preparedness for procedure		x	1	Rassin, Gutman and Silner 2004
Increase privacy and control	Provide areas for privacy within adolescents' patient rooms			Alleviated fears of interruption		x	1	Hutton 2002
	Provide space for companionship and camaraderie in adolescents' patient rooms			Increased satisfaction		x	1	Hutton 2003
	Provide private bathrooms within patient rooms			Alleviated embarrassment		x	1	Hutton 2003
				Increased satisfaction		x	1	Hutton 2003
	Consider a variety of rooming arrangements			Increased satisfaction		x	1	Miller, Friedman and Coupey 1998
	Provide single patient rooms			Increased privacy		x	4	White 2003; Joseph 2006; Landro 2006; Ulrich et al. 2004

APPENDIX | TABLE A: DESIGN CONCEPTS AND ASSOCIATED OUTCOMES | 57

Literature Review Contents	Design Concept Found Within Section of Literature Review	Staff Outcome	Family Outcome	Patient Outcome	Negative Impact	Positive Impact	# of Studies	References Cited
Increase privacy and control	Provide single patient rooms			Increased individuality		x	4	White 2003; Joseph 2006; Landro 2006; Ulrich et al. 2004
				Encouraged family involvement		x	4	White 2003; Joseph 2006; Landro 2006; Ulrich et al. 2004
			Provided opportunity for personalization			x	4	White 2003; Joseph 2006; Landro 2006; Ulrich et al. 2004
		Increased communication from patient to staff		Increased quality of communication from staff to patient		x	3	Joseph 2006; Landro 2006; Ulrich et al. 2004
			Enhanced accommodations			x	3	Joseph 2006; Landro 2006; Ulrich et al. 2004
		Reduced noise	Reduced noise	Reduced noise		x	3	Joseph 2006; Landro 2006; Ulrich et al. 2004
				Reduced infection rates		x	3	Joseph 2006; Landro 2006; Ulrich et al. 2004
		Increased satisfaction	Increased satisfaction	Increased satisfaction		x	3	Joseph 2006; Landro 2006; Ulrich et al. 2004
	Provide single patient rooms in a NICU			Promoted consistent level of appropriate lighting for care delivered		x	1	White 2003
				Promoted consistent level of appropriate sound for care delivered		x	1	White 2003
			Encouraged participation in care			x	1	Bowie et al. 2003
			Increased satisfaction			x	1	Schoenbeck 2006

APPENDIX | TABLE A: DESIGN CONCEPTS AND ASSOCIATED OUTCOMES

Literature Review Contents	Design Concept Found Within Section of Literature Review	Staff Outcome	Family Outcome	Patient Outcome	Negative Impact	Positive Impact	# of Studies	References Cited
Maximize family visitation and participation in care	Provide area for spiritual support		Promoted family involvement in care			x	1	Davidson et al. 2007
	Maximize staff education		Promoted family involvement in care			x	1	Davidson et al. 2007
	Ensure family presence at rounds and resuscitation		Promoted family involvement in care			x	1	Davidson et al. 2007
	Supply family friendly signage		Promoted family involvement in care			x	1	Davidson et al. 2007
	Promote way finding capabilities		Promoted family involvement in care			x	1	Davidson et al. 2007
	Maximize capabilities for sibling visitation			Reduced negative behavior		x	6	Pelander and Leino-Kilpi 2004; Davidson et al. 2007; Moore et al. 2003; Griffin 2003; Lewis et al. 1991; Giacoia, Rutledge and West 1985
			Increased knowledge about ill sibling			x	6	Pelander and Leino-Kilpi 2004; Davidson et al. 2007; Moore et al. 2003; Griffin 2003; Lewis et al. 1991; Giacoia, Rutledge and West 1985
Increase patient and family satisfaction	Provide large patient rooms to accommodate play activities		Increased satisfaction	Increased satisfaction		x	4	Carney et al. 2003; Ayako et al. 2002; Kieffer and Vaughn 1981; Hutton 2002
	Provide entertainment options (videos, interactive communication systems)			Reduced boredom		x	4	Carney et al. 2003; Ayako et al. 2002; Kieffer and Vaughn 1981; Hutton 2002
	Design for a balance between privacy and social interaction		Increased satisfaction	Increased satisfaction		x	1	Mulhall, Kelly and Pearce 2004
	Establish areas with programmed amenities (music instruments, pool tables, art studio)		Reduced the feeling of being in a hospital	Reduced the feeling of being in a hospital		x	1	Mulhall, Kelly and Pearce 2004
	Maximize interior design aesthetics		Increased positive environmental appraisals	Increased positive environmental appraisals		x	2	Leather, Beale et al. 2003; Harris, McBride et al. 2002

APPENDIX | TABLE A: DESIGN CONCEPTS AND ASSOCIATED OUTCOMES | 59

Literature Review Contents	Design Concept Found Within Section of Literature Review	Staff Outcome	Family Outcome	Patient Outcome	Negative Impact	Positive Impact	# of Studies	References Cited
Increase patient and family satisfaction	Maximize interior design aesthetics		Improved satisfaction	Improved satisfaction		x	2	Leather, Beale, et al. 2003; Harris, McBride et al. 2002
			Improved mood	Improved mood		x	2	Leather, Beale, et al. 2003; Harris, McBride et al. 2002
				Altered physiological state		x	2	Leather, Beale, et al. 2003; Harris, McBride et al. 2002
	Design environment which facilitates connection to the outside world		Improved satisfaction	Improved satisfaction		x	1	Fowler, MacRae et al. 1999
	Design environment that provides a connection to staff and caregivers		Improved satisfaction	Improved satisfaction		x	1	Fowler, MacRae et al. 1999
	Design environment that is conducive to a sense of well-being		Improved satisfaction	Improved satisfaction		x	1	Fowler, MacRae et al. 1999
	Provide a garden on site		Improved satisfaction	Improved satisfaction		x	1	Sherman et al. 2005
			Increased perception of restoration and healing	Increased perception of restoration and healing		x	1	Sherman et al. 2005

PROMOTING SAFETY THROUGH DESIGN

Promoting patient safety

Literature Review Contents	Design Concept Found Within Section of Literature Review	Staff Outcome	Family Outcome	Patient Outcome	Negative Impact	Positive Impact	# of Studies	References Cited
Reduce nosocomial infections	Consider environmental transmission routes (air, surface, water) in planning and design	Reduced hospital-acquired infections	Reduced hospital-acquired infections	Reduced hospital-acquired infections		x	1	Joseph 2006
	Maintain hospital ventilation systems to prevent malfunction and contamination	Reduced spread of airborne infections	Reduced spread of airborne infections	Reduced spread of airborne infections		x	3	Kumari et al. 1998; Lutz et al. 2003; McDonald et al. 1998
	Lower room and unit occupancies			Reduced nosocomial infection rates		x	2	Ulrich 2004; Archibald et al. 1997

APPENDIX | TABLE A: DESIGN CONCEPTS AND ASSOCIATED OUTCOMES

Literature Review Contents	Design Concept Found Within Section of Literature Review	Staff Outcome	Family Outcome	Patient Outcome	Negative Impact	Positive Impact	# of Studies	References Cited
Reduce nosocomial infections	Design environments to increase hand washing compliance	Reduced contact transmission infections (patient to staff)		Reduced contact transmission infections (staff to patient)		x	6	Cohen et al. 2003; Hofer et al. 2007; Larson, Albrecht and O'Keefe 2005; Ulrich 2004; Chaberny et al. 2003; Larson 1988
	Maintain sanitation on all children's toys			Reduced nosocomial infection rates		x	2	Avila-Aguero et al. 2004; Buttery et al. 1999
	Design visible and conveniently accessible hand washing sinks and alcohol-based gel dispensers	Increased hand washing compliance				x	2	Joseph 2006; Ulrich et al. 2004
	Maintain sanitation on all water systems and point-of-use water fixtures	Reduced nosocomial infections from waterborne pathogens	Reduced nosocomial infections from waterborne pathogens	Reduced nosocomial infections from waterborne pathogens		x	2	Joseph 2006; Ulrich et al. 2004
	Install barrier precautions during construction and renovation activities	Reduced nosocomial infections from airborne pathogens	Reduced nosocomial infections from airborne pathogens	Reduced nosocomial infections from airborne pathogens		x	2	Joseph 2006; Ulrich et al. 2004
Support communication between patients, families and staff	Design environments to encourage communication between staff members	Prevented replication of efforts				x	3	McCarthy and Blumenthal 2006; Uhlig 2002; Uhlig et al. 2002
		Prevented errors and operational failures				x	3	McCarthy and Blumenthal 2006; Uhlig 2002; Uhlig et al. 2002
	Design environments to support entire care team's presence at bedside	Increased satisfaction		Increased satisfaction		x	3	Uhlig, Brown, Nason, Camelio and Kendall 2002; McCarthy and Blumenthal 2006; Alton et al. 2006
				Reduced mortality rates		x	1	Uhlig, Brown, Nason, Camelio and Kendall 2002
	Increase family space within examination rooms		Increased family participation			x	1	Eckle and MacLean 2001
	Design a variety of spaces for interactive team work	Increased communication and interaction	Increased communication and interaction			x	1	Becker 2007
	Provide visual connections for information seeking and interaction	Increased communication and interaction	Increased communication and interaction			x	1	Becker 2007
	Design flexible work spaces	Increased communication and interaction				x	1	Becker 2007
	Design a smaller unit size	Fostered interaction				x	1	Becker 2007

APPENDIX | TABLE A: DESIGN CONCEPTS AND ASSOCIATED OUTCOMES | 61

Literature Review Contents	Design Concept Found Within Section of Literature Review	Staff Outcome	Family Outcome	Patient Outcome	Negative Impact	Positive Impact	# of Studies	References Cited
Support communication between patients, families and staff	Provide neutral spaces	Minimized professional and status hierarchies				x	1	Becker 2007
Reduce medical errors	Reduce high noise levels	Minimized point of service errors				x	5	Reiling et al. 2004; Buchanan et al. 1991; Tucker and Spear 2006; Flynn et al. 1999; Flynn et al. 1996
	Minimize chaotic environments; Reduce frequent distractions and interruptions	Reduced medical errors				x	4	Buchanan et al. 1991; Tucker and Spear 2006; Flynn et al. 1999; Flynn et al. 1996
	Provide adequate light levels for visual tasks	Reduced medical errors				x	4	Buchanan et al. 1991; Tucker and Spear 2006; Flynn et al. 1999; Flynn et al. 1996
Reduce patient transfers	Equip patient rooms with acuity adaptable headwalls			Decreased patient transfers		x	2	Hendrich, Fay and Sorrells 2004; Hendrich and Lee 2005
		Reduced medical errors				x	2	Hendrich, Fay and Sorrells 2004; Hendrich and Lee 2005
				Reduced falls		x	2	Hendrich, Fay and Sorrells 2004; Hendrich and Lee 2005
Reduce falls and injuries	Consider possible hazards from beds and cribs			Reduced falls		x	2	Warda 2005; Buick 2007
	Do not design bedrails that cause entrapment			Reduced falls		x	2	Hignett and Masud 2006; Rice and Nelson 2005
	Provide decentralized nurse stations	Increased visibility to patient				x	1	Hendrich et al. 2003
				Reduced falls		x	1	Hendrich et al. 2003
	Consider wooden sub-floors in lieu of concrete sub-floors			Reduced risk of fracture from fall		x	1	Simpson 2004
	Consider type of flooring-vinyl			Reduced falls		x	1	Donald 2000
	Consider type of flooring-carpet			Reduced injury contributed from fall		x	1	Healy 2004

APPENDIX | TABLE A: DESIGN CONCEPTS AND ASSOCIATED OUTCOMES

Literature Review Contents	Design Concept Found Within Section of Literature Review	Staff Outcome	Family Outcome	Patient Outcome	Negative Impact	Positive Impact	# of Studies	References Cited
Promoting staff safety	Conduct ergonomic evaluations of work areas	Reduced neck and back problems				x	1	Gerbrands et al. 2004
	Provide exposure to bright light during night shift	Improved mood				x	1	Leppamaki et al. 2003
		Improved sleep				x	1	Leppamaki et al. 2003
		Adapted circadian rhythms				x	6	Baehr, Fogg and Eastman 1999; Boivin and James 2002; Crowley et al. 2003; Horowitz et al. 2001; Iwata, Ichii and Egashira 1997; Leppamaki et al. 2003
	Improve air quality	Reduced hospital-acquired infections				x	1	Joseph 2007
	Design visible and conveniently accessible hand washing sinks and alcohol-based gel dispensers	Reduced hospital-acquired infections				x	1	Joseph 2007

INCREASE STAFF EFFECTIVENESS IN PROVIDING CARE THROUGH DESIGN

Literature Review Contents	Design Concept Found Within Section of Literature Review	Staff Outcome	Family Outcome	Patient Outcome	Negative Impact	Positive Impact	# of Studies	References Cited
Decrease staff stress	Consider the design of environments around routine events (coming to work, shift change, presenting rounds) to reduce stress	Reduced stress				x	1	Fischer et al. 2000
	Improve acoustical conditions on unit and in patient room	Reduced emotional exhaustion				x	2	Topf and Dillon 1988; Parsons and Hartig 2000
		Reduced work interference				x	3	Joseph 2006; Morrison et al. 2003; Bayo, Garcia and Garcia 1995
		Reduced burnout				x	1	Topf and Dillon 1988
				Improved patient comfort		x	1	Bayo, Garcia and Garcia 1995
				Improved patient recovery		x	1	Bayo, Garcia and Garcia 1995
		Reduced reported pressure and strain				x	2	Blomkvist et al. 2005; Parsons and Hartig 2000

APPENDIX | TABLE A: DESIGN CONCEPTS AND ASSOCIATED OUTCOMES | 63

Literature Review Contents	Design Concept Found Within Section of Literature Review	Staff Outcome	Family Outcome	Patient Outcome	Negative Impact	Positive Impact	# of Studies	References Cited
Decrease staff stress	Improve acoustical conditions on unit and in patient room	Reduced fatigue				x	1	Bailey and Timmons 2005
		Reduced irritability				x	1	Bailey and Timmons 2005
		Reduced anxiety				x	1	Bailey and Timmons 2005
		Reduced impaired judgment				x	1	Bailey and Timmons 2005
		Improved concentration				x	1	Bailey and Timmons 2005
	Provide access to nature through gardens	Increased satisfaction				x	2	Ulrich et al. 2004; Cooper-Marcus and Barnes 1995
		Fostered social support				x	2	Ulrich et al. 2004; Cooper-Marcus and Barnes 1995
		Increased recuperation from stressful clinical situations				x	2	Ulrich et al. 2004; Cooper-Marcus and Barnes 1995
			Increased patient-visitor interaction	Increased patient-visitor interaction		x	1	Cooper-Marcus 2005
			Increased positive mood	Increased positive mood		x	1	Ulrich et al. 2004
			Reduced stress	Reduced stress		x	1	Ulrich et al. 2004
		Reduced emotional distress	Reduced emotional distress	Reduced emotional distress		x	1	Sherman et al. 2005
				Reduced pain		x	1	Sherman et al. 2005
	Consider visibility, accessibility and familiarity within garden design	Increased garden use	Increased garden use	Increased garden use		x	1	Cooper-Marcus 2005

APPENDIX | TABLE A: DESIGN CONCEPTS AND ASSOCIATED OUTCOMES

Literature Review Contents	Design Concept Found Within Section of Literature Review	Staff Outcome	Family Outcome	Patient Outcome	Negative Impact	Positive Impact	# of Studies	References Cited
Decrease staff stress	Promote quiet sound environment within garden	Increased garden use	Increased garden use	Increased garden use		x	1	Cooper-Marcus 2005
	Provide areas for comfort within garden	Increased garden use	Increased garden use	Increased garden use		x	1	Cooper-Marcus 2005
	Include unambiguously positive art within garden	Increased garden use	Increased garden use	Increased garden use		x	1	Cooper-Marcus 2005
	Provide view to nature	Reduced acute stress				x	1	Pati and Barach (in review)
Increase staff satisfaction	Design smaller units	Increased communication				x	1	Walsh, McCullough and White 2006
		Promoted staff education				x	1	Walsh, McCullough and White 2006
		Minimized quality improvement challenges				x	1	Walsh, McCullough and White 2006
	Design private room NICU	Decreased interaction among team members			x		1	Schoenbeck 2006
		Decreased patient visibility			x		1	Schoenbeck 2006
			Improved interaction with family members			x	1	Schoenbeck 2006
	Maximize interior design aesthetics	Increased level of confidence with regard to environment				x	1	Judkins 2003
		Increased satisfaction				x	1	Judkins 2003
		Increased coworker relationship satisfaction				x	1	Varni et al. 2004
	Incorporate natural light	Increased satisfaction				x	1	Altimier 2004
		Improved morale				x	1	Altimier 2004
		Improved retention				x	1	Altimier 2004

APPENDIX | **TABLE A: DESIGN CONCEPTS AND ASSOCIATED OUTCOMES** | 65

Literature Review Contents	Design Concept Found Within Section of Literature Review	Staff Outcome	Family Outcome	Patient Outcome	Negative Impact	Positive Impact	# of Studies	References Cited
Increase staff satisfaction	Incorporate views of nature	Increased satisfaction				x	1	Altimier 2004
		Improved morale				x	1	Altimier 2004
		Improved retention				x	1	Altimier 2004
	Include soothing colors within the environment	Increased satisfaction				x	1	Altimier 2004
		Improved morale				x	1	Altimier 2004
		Improved retention				x	1	Altimier 2004
	Offer therapeutic sounds within the environment	Increased satisfaction				x	1	Altimier 2004
		Improved morale				x	1	Altimier 2004
		Improved retention				x	1	Altimier 2004
	Maximize storage space; include wheelchair storage within each patient room	Increased satisfaction				x	1	Varni et al. 2004
	Include a staff break room within program and plan	Increased satisfaction				x	1	Varni et al. 2004
	Design larger bathrooms with showers	Increased satisfaction				x	1	Varni et al. 2004
	Design larger activity spaces	Increased satisfaction				x	1	Varni et al. 2004
	Include a dining room within program and plan	Increased satisfaction				x	1	Varni et al. 2004
	Design a large outdoor recreation area	Increased satisfaction				x	1	Varni et al. 2004

… | APPENDIX | TABLE A: DESIGN CONCEPTS AND ASSOCIATED OUTCOMES

Literature Review Contents	Design Concept Found Within Section of Literature Review	Staff Outcome	Family Outcome	Patient Outcome	Negative Impact	Positive Impact	# of Studies	References Cited
Increase staff effectiveness and efficiency	Consider distances between patient rooms, nurses stations and supply areas when designing the layout of the unit	Reduced fatigue				x	1	Joseph 2007
		Increased time spent with patient		Increased patient-staff time		x	5	Joseph 2007; Shepley 2002; Shepley and Davies 2003; Sturdavant 1960; Trites, Galbraith, Sturdavant and Leckwart 1970
		Reduced time spent walking				x	1	Joseph 2007
			Improved family interaction			x	4	Shepley 2002; Shepley and Davies 2003; Sturdavant 1960; Trites, Galbraith, Sturdavant and Leckwart 1970
	Increase light levels for task performance	Reduced rate of medication dispensing errors				x	1	Buchanan et al. 1991
		Improved task performance				x	2	Boyce, Hunter and Howlett 2003; Buchanan et al. 1991

Article Analysis Methodology

Articles were assessed individually for quality, rigor and relevance to the study at hand. The studies were classified as one of the following: experimental, quasi experimental, controlled observational studies (cohort or case control), observational studies (without control groups, surveys, case studies) and expert opinion. Within each of these categories, studies were rated as good, fair or poor using the methodology (Ulrich et al., In Press) in Table 2. Additionally, population and sample size of the study were assessed as well as confounding variables and tools were identified.

TABLE B: Article Analysis Methodology (Ulrich et al., In Press)

A study must meet all of the applicable criteria to receive a "good" rating. A study should be rated as "fair" if most of the criteria are met, and "poor" if most are not met or if is the study has a fatal flaw.

	YES	NO
I. EXPERIMENTAL STUDIES		
Was the assignment to the treatment groups really random?		
• Adequate approaches to sequence generation		
• Computer-generated random numbers		
• Random numbers tables		
• Inadequate approaches to sequence generation		
• Use of alternation, case record numbers, birth dates or week days		
• Was the treatment allocation concealed?		
Adequate approaches to concealment of randomization		
• Centralized or pharmacy-controlled randomization		
• Serially-numbered identical containers		
• On-site computer based system with a randomization sequence that is not readable until allocation		
• Other approaches with robust methods to prevent foreknowledge of the allocation sequence to clinicians and patients		
Inadequate approaches to concealment of randomization		
• Use of alternation, case record numbers, birth dates or week days		
• Open random numbers lists		
• Serially numbered envelopes (even sealed opaque envelopes can be subject to manipulation)		
Were the groups similar at baseline in terms of health?		
Were the groups treated similarly with the exception of the intervention?		
Were the eligibility criteria specified?		
Were outcome assessors blinded to the treatment allocation?		
Was the care provider blinded?		
Was the patient blinded?		
Were alternate hypotheses effectively ruled out?		
II. QUASI-EXPERIMENTAL STUDIES		
Was the treatment allocation concealed?		
Adequate approaches to concealment of randomization		
• Centralized or pharmacy-controlled randomization		
• Serially-numbered identical containers		
• On-site computer based system with a randomization sequence that is not readable until allocation		
Other approaches with robust methods to prevent foreknowledge of the allocation sequence to clinicians and patients		

	YES	NO
Inadequate approaches to concealment of randomization		
• Use of alternation, case record numbers, birth dates or week days		
• Open random numbers lists		
• Serially numbered envelopes (even sealed opaque envelopes can be subject to manipulation)		
Were the groups similar at baseline in terms of health?		
Were the groups treated similarly with the exception of the intervention?		
Were the eligibility criteria specified?		
Were outcome assessors blinded to the treatment allocation?		
Was the care provider blinded?		
Was the patient blinded?		
Were alternate hypotheses effectively ruled out?		
III. (A) CONTROLLED OBSERVATIONAL STUDIES: COHORT STUDIES		
Is there sufficient description of the groups and additional variables that might impact the outcomes?		
Were the groups comparable on all important confounding factors?		
Was there adequate adjustment for the effects of these confounding variables?		
Was outcome assessment blind to exposure status?		
Was follow-up long enough for the outcomes to occur?		
Were drop-out rates and reasons for drop-out similar across intervention and unexposed groups?		
III. (B) CONTROLLED OBSERVATIONAL STUDIES: CASE CONTROL STUDIES		
Is the case definition explicit?		
Has the disease state (or dependent measure) of the cases been reliably assessed and validated?		
Were the controls randomly selected from the source of population of the cases?		
How comparable are the cases and controls with respect to potential confounding factors?		
Were interventions and other exposures assessed in the same way for cases and controls?		
Were the non-response rates and reasons for non-response the same in both groups?		
Is it possible that over-matching has occurred in that cases and controls were matched on factors related to exposure?		
IV. OBSERVATIONAL STUDIES WITHOUT CONTROL GROUPS, SINGLE CASE STUDY, SURVEYS		
Is the study based on a representative sample selected from a relevant population?		
Are the criteria for inclusion explicit?		
Did all individuals enter the survey at a similar point in their disease progression, length of stay, time on the job or other relevant measure?		
Was follow-up long enough for important events to occur?		
Were outcomes assessed using objective criteria or was blinding used?		
V. EXPERT OPINION		
Does the author have an apparent or stated conflict-of-interest with the results (e.g. is a sales person for the product)?		
Is this a collaborative effort or just one person's opinion?		
Does the author have substantial hands-on experience in the matter?		

APPENDIX | TABLE C: ARTICLE ANALYSIS SAMPLE | 69

Study	Type of Study: Experimental	Quasi experimental	Controlled observational	Observ., no control groups	Expert opinion, consensus	Research Methods	Population	Sample Size	Tools Used	Limitations	Major Findings	Criteria Guide
Al-Samsam, R. and O. Cullen (2005). "Sleep and adverse environmental factors in sedated mechanically ventilated pediatric intensive care patients." Pediatric Critical Care Medicine 6(5): 562-567.				x		The researchers looked at sound level (using a microphone), staff interventions (any tactile stimulation), sleep (monitored with a variety of technologies). Patients were monitored for 24 hrs, which was split into day (7 am- 7 pm) and night (7 pm to 7 am).	PICU patients, greater than 3 months of age, in the PICU for more than 24 hours, anticipation of continued ventilation, mean age of 9 months, all were ventilated and sedated.	11	Quest Technologies, Model Q-300 microphone; tactile stimulation, Respironics PSG Alice 4	The sleep patterns could be a result of the sedative drugs and not any environmental condition; no causality determined. No control group, small number of patients, mixed diagnoses, only one point in PICU stay.	Sound: Day was significantly louder than night. Staff: There was no significant difference between night and day. Sleep: Patients were awake 40 times during the night. The amount of REM was much lower than comparison healthy children, but similar to adult ICU patients.	Fair
American Art Resources & Memorial Hermann Hospital (In Review). "Pediatric Art Preferences."				x		Patients were asked to rate pictures, starting with the current picture on their wall, followed with a variety of other pictures. Pictures were chosen from the categories of waterscapes, landscapes, flowers and figurative. Overall and between group comparisons were made.	Patients in the pediatric ward of a children's hospital. The children were split into the three developmental stages identified by Piaget.	In order to get 80% power, there were 13 5-6 yr olds, 27 7-10 yr olds, and 24 11-17 year olds. Total: 64.	Completed a survey on pictures, rated them using a feeling scale, whether or not they would want it in their room and a faces scale.	Though the study indicates that statistical tools were used, they do not identify significance or the results.	Bright colors, engaging themes and nature content was consistently rated high, realistic nature with bright colors, water and friendly wildlife were also good. There are differences between the three stages. Child art was better for younger than older children. Comic/iconic images were different for age groups.	Fair
Archibald, L. K., M. L. Manning, et al. (1997). "Patient density, nurse-to-patient ratio and nosocomial infection risk in a pediatric cardiac intensive care unit." The Pediatric Infectious Disease Journal 16(11): 1045-8.				x		Monthly nursing hours, patient days and nosocomial infections for one year were collected from medical records. Correlational analysis was conducted to find the relation between patient density, nurse-to-patient ratio, nosocomial infection rates.	Monthly nursing hours, patient days and nosocomial infections for one year in a PICU	782 admissions in 12 months	Medical records	Correlational analysis. Cause-effect relation cannot be justified.	Monthly nosocomial infection rates were positively associated with patient days and negatively associated with nursing hour-to-patient day ratio.	Fair

APPENDIX | TABLE C: ARTICLE ANALYSIS SAMPLE

Study	Type of Study	Research Methods	Population	Sample Size	Tools Used	Limitations	Major Findings	Criteria Guide
Arnon, S., A. Shapsa, et al. (2006). "Live music is beneficial to preterm infants in the neonatal intensive care unit environment." Birth 33(2): 131-136.	Quasi experimental (x)	Stable infants randomly received live music, recorded music and no music therapy over 3 consecutive days. A control of the environment noise level was imposed. Therapy was delivered for 30 minutes. A questionnaire for parents and medical personnel was delivered.	31 stable infants: post conception age >32 weeks, weight >1,500g, and hearing confirmed by distortion product otoacoustic emissions, no active illness.	31	Heart rate, respiratory rate, oxygen saturation and behavioral assessment recorded		Live music therapy had no significant effect on physiological and behavioral parameters during therapy sessions however it significantly reduced heart rate and improved behavioral score.	Good
Avila-Aguero, M., G. German, et al. (2004). "Toys in a pediatric hospital: Are they a bacterial source?" American Journal of Infection Control 32(5): 287-290.	Controlled observational (x)	Within 48 hours of hospital admission, pediatric patient's toys were swabbed and the cultures were tested for contamination using standard laboratory methods. Then the toys were cleaned and immediately re-cultured. Following cultures were obtained and tested every week until discharge.	Children's toys in a pediatric hospital	70	Laboratory tests	The number of toys tested reduced significantly for the second and the subsequent tests.	All toys were contaminated by at least one pathogenic microorganism. The contamination level decreased after cleaning. Plastic toys were more likely to be contaminated (75%), followed by metallic toys (16%) and other toys (9%).	Fair
Bailey, E. and S. Timmons (2005). "Noise levels in PICU: an evaluative study." Pediatric Nursing 17(10): 22-26.	Observ., no control groups (x)	Literature review, noise level readings every five minutes over a period of 12 hours during both day and night shifts.	PICU patients and staff in 1,300 bed teaching hospital; 600 patients admitted per year		Tenma sound level meter	Staff aware of researcher on site which in turn resulted in a change behavior when researcher was present—Hawthorne effect. PICU had low levels of occupancy.	Observation of the causes of noise in 1 PICU indicated that staff conversation was responsible for most noise.	Fair

APPENDIX | TABLE C: ARTICLE ANALYSIS SAMPLE | 71

Study	Type of Study: Experimental	Quasi experimental	Controlled observational	Observ., no control groups	Expert opinion, consensus	Research Methods	Population	Sample Size	Tools Used	Limitations	Major Findings	Criteria Guide
Battles, H. and L. Wiener (2002). "Starbright World: Effects of an Electronic Network on the Social Environment of Children with Life-Threatening Illnesses." Children's Health Care 31(1): 47-68.	x					Repeated measurements in 8 30-minute playroom sessions: 4 Starbright World (SBW) and 4 normal playrooms. Pediatric patients were randomly assigned to sessions. Questionnaire surveys were conducted for scale measurement.	Pediatric patients (age 8-19 years) participating in outpatient pediatric clinical trials at the National Institutes of Health and their caregivers (parents and staff members)	32 caregiver-child dyads	Ecological Momentary Assessment, State Anger Inventory, Faces Pain Scale, Anxiety Analogue Scale, Depression and Exhaustion Analogue Scales, University of California Loneliness Scale-8, Child Behavior Checklist, child interview, parent survey and staff survey.	Part of the study (on loneliness, problem behavior and willingness to return) used a pre-post design and did not use an experimental design.	Patients reported to be marginally less worried in SBW condition than in the normal playroom condition. SBW condition was related to significantly less loneliness and more willingness to return to the hospital. Parents reported that their children experienced less withdrawn behavior, lower level of anxiety and resistance in returning to the hospital and positive change in mood.	Fair
Bellieni, C. V., G. Buonocore, et al. (2003). "Use of sound-absorbing panel to reduce noisy incubator reverberating effects." Biol Neonate 84(4): 293-6.				x		Compared the sound in the incubator between closed hood, open hood, sound absorbing panel. Looked at reverberating sound.	No actual patients/people were used.	NA	Larson Davis model 2800 class 1 real time analyzer, a Larson Davis 2541 microphone, a Larson Davis model 900B microphone preamplifier, a Larson Davis CA 250 calibrator.	Only technology was used in this study and the results are very mixed and unclear.	The reverberation within the incubator had a significant effect on the noise neonates perceive when in an incubator. The reverberation was significant. Opening the hood or using sound absorbing panels can help.	good
Berens, R. (1999). "Noise in the Pediatric Intensive Care Unit." Journal of Intensive Care Medicine 14(3): 118-129.					x	Literature review	N/A	N/A	N/A	The discussion of environmental change could have been more systematic.	PICU was noisy. Research showed that noise could result in hearing-loss and impairment, excessive stress and disturbed sleep. Noise abatement methods included behavioral change, environmental modification and equipment such as noise canceling devices.	Fair
Bers, M., J. Gonzalez-Heydrich, et al. (2001). "Zora: a pilot virtual community in the pediatric dialysis unit." Medinfo 10(Part 1): 800-804.			x			Ethnographic approach; observations of online and face to face interaction and online analysis, interviews with patients and staff using a 7 point Likert scale, qualitative analysis of videotaped interviews	Pediatric patients with renal disease while undergoing hemodialysis	7 out of 12	Zora, an object-orientated environment implemented using Microsoft's Virtual Worlds research platform	Small sample size	Zora was seen as contributing to positive outcomes however patients reported that using Zora did not help them gain perspective or understanding about their illness. Children utilized Zora as a positive distraction, a method for escape rather than a place to talk about their procedures and illness. The study revealed that utilizing a virtual environment within a dialysis unit was feasible and safe.	Fair

APPENDIX | TABLE C: ARTICLE ANALYSIS SAMPLE

Study	Type of Study	Research Methods	Population	Sample Size	Tools Used	Limitations	Major Findings	Criteria Guide
Blumberg, R. and A. S. Devlin (2006). "Design Issues in Hospitals: The adolescent client." Environment and Behavior 38(3): 293-317.	Observ., no control groups (x)	Survey participants were asked to describe their ideal room, hospital room, and compare adult and children hospital facilities. The findings were then analyzed using statistical and observational methods.	12-14 yr old junior high students, not in hospital, upper middle class-middle class, primarily white, from 4 classrooms	100	Demographics questionnaire, photographic comparison task (looking at pictures of adult and children's hospitals), design questionnaire (part 1 on ideal bedroom, part 2 on ideal hospital room)	Students gave opinions of an idealized hospital environment whether or not they had ever been in a hospital. The survey was administered in a classroom and students were given the opportunity to discuss as a group, which may have impacted their responses.	Adolescents wanted to have family and friends present, colors but no child-related decorations, entertainment, technology, privacy, may or may not want a library, control.	Poor
Bowie, B. H., R. B. Hall, et al. (2003). "Single-room infant care: future trends in special care nursery planning and design." Neonatal Network 22(4): 27-34.	Observ., no control groups (x)	The article described the design process of a special care nursery, including the organization of a multidisciplinary team, space programming, schematic design, environmental design and design development.	A special care nursery	1	Case study (literature review, interview)	Generalizability	The design incorporated the concepts of family centered care, developmentally supportive care and staff work efficiency. Design features included: single bed patient rooms for family participation in the care, noise control (carpeting, separation and acoustical ceiling system), flexible lighting, windows between rooms and electronic devices for patient visibility and monitoring.	Fair
Boyd, J. and M. Hunsberger (1998). "Chronically ill children coping with repeated hospitalizations: their perceptions and suggested interventions." Journal of Pediatric Nursing 13(6): 330-342.	Observ., no control groups (x)	The perspectives and coping strategies of patients in a tertiary pediatric hospital were collected using three techniques: art work, semi-structured interview and journal keeping. All the data were transcribed verbatim for content analysis.	Hospitalized children with chronic conditions	6	Content analysis	Small sample size	Perceived stressors included hospital environment elements, such as noise, lack of privacy. Distraction and familiarity were among the coping strategies. TV, phone, diverse activities, a quiet private room with spaces for a parent, outside view and playroom were preferred by patients.	Fair

APPENDIX | TABLE C: ARTICLE ANALYSIS SAMPLE | 73

Study	Type of Study — Experimental	Quasi experimental	Controlled observational	Observ, no control groups	Expert opinion, consensus	Research Methods	Population	Sample Size	Tools Used	Limitations	Major Findings	Criteria Guide
Brandon, D. H., D. Holditch-Davis, et al. (2002). "Preterm infants born at less than 31 weeks' gestation have improved growth in cycled light compared with continuous near darkness." The Journal of Pediatrics 140(2): 192-199.			x			3 groups received cycled light at different times—from birth, at 32 weeks and 36 weeks. The other times patients received near darkness. There was random assignment to the groups.	Infants born at greater than 31 weeks, 60 infants participated (to reach 93% power), no anomalies, most were non-white, half female.	60	Growth, number of ventilator days and length of stay, hearing, retinopathy of prematurely, covariates	The only power analysis was related to weight, therefore extrapolating on the other parts of the study is difficult because of the lack of power.	Cycled light had short-term advantages over continuous near darkness for infants. Weight: Significantly greater gains for infants receiving cycled light earlier than other patients. Ventilator days and length of stay: no statistical differences, though it did increase for infants who did not receive cycled light earlier. Auditory: Infants who received cycled light earlier had greater loss than those who received it later, but not significant. Retinopathy development: Near darkness group had more severe retinopathy earlier, but not significant.	Good
Bremmer, P., J. Byers, et al. (2003). "Noise and the premature infant: Physiological effects and practice implications." Journal of Obstetric, Gynecologic, and Neonatal Nursing 32(4): 447-454.				x		Literature review exploring the premature infant's developing acoustic ability in relation to the environment of the NICU	N/A	N/A	Literature review	Authors noted limited research conducted on noise and the premature infant.	Excessive auditory stimuli negatively affected the premature infant by increasing heart rate, blood pressure and respiratory rate, and decreasing oxygen saturation. Several studies documented a direct cause and effect relationship between personnel conversation and increased noise levels in the NICU. Article included clinical interventions to decrease noise in the NICU.	Good
Brokstein, R., S. Cohen, et al. (2002). "Starbright World and Psychological Adjustment in Children with Cancer: A clinical series." Children's Health Care 31(1): 29-45.				x		Qualitative case studies of the interaction of pediatric cancer patients with a computer system. The data were collected through observation and the use of computer system records.	Pediatric cancer patients (10-17 yr olds)	4	Observation and the use of computer system data	No comparisons. Small sample size	The computer system provided a platform for receiving information about diseases and social support from others. It appeared to be well accepted by the patients.	Fair

APPENDIX | TABLE C: ARTICLE ANALYSIS SAMPLE

Study	Type of Study (Experimental / Quasi experimental / Controlled observational / Observ, no control groups / Expert opinion, consensus)	Research Methods	Population	Sample Size	Tools Used	Limitations	Major Findings	Criteria Guide
Brown, B., H. Wright, et al. (1997). "A post-occupancy evaluation of way finding in a pediatric hospital: Research findings and implications for instruction." Journal of Architectural & Planning Research 14(1): 35-51.	Observ, no control groups: x	Interviews with staff members and visitors, diaries kept by staff, traces (handmade signs), observation, cognitive maps	Visitors, staff and patients at a children's hospital	Interviews: 66 staff and 47 visitors; diaries: 46 staff summaries; 193 observed and 13 visitors tracked; plans from 11 school age and toddler patients and 3 parents	Interviews, photographs, observation, diaries		Environmental cues were used much more by inpatient than outpatient visitors. Staff perceived spending a lot of time directing people through the hospital and made recommendations for improvement, including parking lot distinction, aesthetic goals sometimes inhibited effective way finding, more PICU direction and more environmental cues should be created.	Good
Buttery, J., S. Alabaster, et al. (1998). "Multiresistant psuedomonas aeruginosa outbreak in a pediatric oncology ward related to bath toys." Pediatric Infectious Disease Journal 17(6): 509-513.	Controlled observational: x	After an outbreak of P. aeruginosa, all wet areas in a pediatric oncology unit were sampled and tested for contamination. Laboratory tests were performed on patient and environmental isolates. A case-control study was conducted to detect possible routes of the infection and outbreak.	Infected patients (cases) and 3 non-infected patients (controls) matching each infected patient on underlying disease	8 cases plus 24 controls	Environmental sampling, laboratory tests	Retrospective study. The study did not exclude the possibility of infectious transmission through other modes, such as direct contact transmission.	Bath toys and toy box water were contaminated. The isolates from the 8 cases, toys and toy box water were identical. Controlled for age and underlying disease, there was a marginally significant relation between infection and the use of bath toys.	Fair

APPENDIX | TABLE C: ARTICLE ANALYSIS SAMPLE | 75

Study	Type of Study: Experimental	Quasi experimental	Controlled observational	Observ., no control groups	Expert opinion, consensus	Research Methods	Population	Sample Size	Tools Used	Limitations	Major Findings	Criteria Guide
Byers, J. F., W. R. Waugh, et al. (2006). "Sound level exposure of high-risk infants in different environmental conditions." Neonatal Network: NN 25(1): 25-32.						STUDY 1: Convenience sample, comparison between a control and renovated NICU, the study looked at the difference between a "developmental NICU" and a regular NICU. The renovated NICU had such changes as sound-absorbing materials in the ceiling, flooring and wall panels, privacy curtains, lower light levels and special classes for the nurses. STUDY 2: Assessed the sound of equipment: therapy pumps, monitors, respiratory therapy equipment and alarms.	STUDY 1: Convenience sample, NICU infants, 78 bed NICU; STUDY 2: incubators	STUDY 1: 134; STUDY 2: once	Quest Technologies' Model 2900 sound level meter, sound levels were measuring 1 day per month for 6 months, measured near the ear of a NICU infant.	The study looked at many variables at once — cannot tell what was the most effective intervention. The study was descriptive — no cause and effect. The incubator was slightly open in order to get the microphone near the ear of the infant.	The renovated NICU was significantly quieter than the regular. However, both NICUs were above the recommended noise level. There was a slight decrease in the noise of the newer incubators.	Fair
Cohen, B., L. Saiman, et al. (2003). "Factors associated with hand hygiene practices in two neonatal intensive care units." Pediatric Infectious Diseases Journal 22(6): 494-9.			x			Factors associated with hand hygiene practices were examined. Hand hygiene practices in 2 NICUs were compared to determine the influence of hand hygiene products.	1,472 patient care touches (by nurse, visitors and physicians) observed in 38 observation periods.	1,472	Observation	Other differences between the two NICUs might contribute to the difference in hand hygiene.	The average number of direct touches by staff members with cleaned hands was higher in the NICU using alcohol-based hand rubs than in the NICU using antimicrobial soap.	Fair
Davidson, J. E., K. Powers, et al. (2006). "Clinical practice guidelines for support of the family in the patient-centered intensive care unit: American College of Critical Care Medicine Task Force 2004-2005." Critical Care Medicine 35(2): 605-622.					x	Task force of experts in critical care practice reviewed published literature. Studies were scored according to the Cochrane methodology. Where evidence did not exist, consensus was derived from expert opinion.	N/A	N/A	Cochrane library, Cinahl, MedLine	Level of evidence in most articles indicated a need for further research.	300 related studies were reviewed. 43 recommendations were presented to include: endorsement of a shared decision-making model, early and repeated care conferencing to reduce family stress and improve consistency in communication, spiritual support, staff education, family presence at rounds and resuscitation, open flexible visitation, way-finding, family friendly signage and family support before, during and after death.	Good

APPENDIX | TABLE C: ARTICLE ANALYSIS SAMPLE

Study	Type of Study (Experimental / Quasi experimental / Controlled observational / Observ., no control groups / Expert opinion, consensus)	Research Methods	Population	Sample Size	Tools Used	Limitations	Major Findings	Criteria Guide
Eckle, N. and S. MacLean (2001). "Assessment of family-centered care policies and practices for pediatric patients in nine US emergency departments." Journal of Emergency Nursing 27(3): 238-245.	Observ., no control groups (x)	The Family Centered Care Self-assessment Inventory was used to evaluate family centered care in nine emergency departments (EDs). Qualitative interviews were conducted to identify areas of strength and weakness.	Pediatric emergency departments and general emergency departments serving adults and pediatric patients	9 (5 pediatric and 4 general)	Family Centered Care Self-assessment Inventory	No comparison	External signage clearly indicated the location of ED entrance. Internal signage was more variable. Dual language signs were limited. Amenities such as phones, vendor machines, ATMs, spaces for diaper-changing and breast-feeding were provided. However, the seating configuration in waiting area did not meet the special needs of children and adults. In some EDs, patients were separated visually but not acoustically. Private rooms provided more spaces for families than curtained areas.	Fair
Eisert, D., L. Kulka, et al. (1988). "Facilitating Play in Hospitalized Handicapped Children: The Design of a Therapeutic Play Environment." Child Health Care 16(3): 201-208.	Controlled observational (x)	The play behaviors of handicapped patients in a pediatric rehabilitation hospital before and after the construction of a play structure were observed and compared.	Handicapped patients in a pediatric rehabilitation hospital	22 patients in the pretest sample, 31 in the posttest sample.	Behavior coding	Generalizability	Special considerations in the design of the play structure included: controlling unnecessary sources of stimulation, encouraging exploration and allowing for individual abilities. There was significant increase in total play behavior, symbolic play and partial play after the construction of the new play structure. Unoccupied wandering decreased.	Fair
Fels, D. I., J. K. Waalen, et al. "Telepresence under exceptional circumstances: enriching the connection to school for sick children."	Observ., no control groups (x)	3 case studies were carried out on the effects of a new computer system on sick children. The usage of the system and perceptions of students, teachers, parents and medical staff were collected by a video analysis program, questionnaire and interview.	Sick children with renal failure or kidney transplant	3	Video analysis program, questionnaire, interview	Generalizability	Sick students in remote locations were able to engage in the same tasks as their classmates, to make positive contributions and to communicate. The system played a role in enhancing a feel of real classroom presence and behavior for the sick children.	Fair

APPENDIX | TABLE C: ARTICLE ANALYSIS SAMPLE | 77

Study	Type of Study					Research Methods	Population	Sample Size	Tools Used	Limitations	Major Findings	Criteria Guide
	Experimental	Quasi experimental	Controlled observational	Observ., no control groups	Expert opinion, consensus							
Gariepy, N. and N. Howe (2003). "The therapeutic power of play: examining the play of young children with leukemia." Child: Care, Health and Development 29(6): 523-537.			x			The effects of play on children with leukemia (3-5 yr olds) were compared with healthy children.	11 pediatric patient with leukemia from an oncology clinic and 11 healthy children from a day care center	22	Early Childhood Environment Rating Scale, Self-Distress Measure, Stress Inventory	Small sample size	Children with leukemia engaged in more repetitive play activities, fewer total play behaviors, less parallel, group and dramatic play than healthy children. For children with leukemia, play was associated with "being happy".	Fair
Gershon, J., E. Zimand, et al. (2003). "Use of virtual reality as a distracter for painful procedures in a patient with pediatric cancer: a case study." Cyberpsychology & Behavior 6(6): 657-61.						A single subject, repeated measures (A-B-C-A) design was used. A patient undergoing invasive procedures was able to use a virtual reality (VR) game to avert anxiety. First there was no intervention, then the game on a television, then the VR, then no intervention again. The game was an interactive guerilla game designed for the Zoo.	8 yr old, Caucasian male, acute lymphocytic leukemia, diagnosed 2 yrs prior, parental presence for all procedures	1	Multidimensional Anxiety Scale for Children, Visual Analogue Scale, Child Behavior Checklist, pulse rate monitoring, Children's Hospital of Eastern Ontario Pain Scale, Virtual Gorilla program	The posttest was much lower than the baseline; need to determine what the conditioning has an effect on.	Pain lowest during condition C; patient's anxiety ratings were lowest during condition B- most likely due to patient's ability to observe what was going on or understand the abstract concept of anxiety (pain was still lowest during condition C).	Good
Giacoia, G. P., D. Rutledge, et al. (1985). "Factors affecting visitation of sick newborns." Clinical Pediatrics 24(5): 259-262.				x		Questionnaire surveys and interviews were conducted with the parents of sick newborns admitted to a NICU were interviewed. The data were divided into 2 groups according to the residential locations: residents from the metropolitan area and from out-of-town. The visitation patterns of these 2 groups were compared.	Parents of sick newborns admitted to a NICU	167 admissions	Questionnaire survey	No control of confounding factors	Parents in the out-of-town group visited less often, made fewer telephone inquiries and earned a lower salary. The average cost of travel from home to hospital was higher for the out-of-town group. Visitation frequency was related to social status. Factors limiting visitation included: care of other children, work demands, travel cost and distance.	Fair

APPENDIX | TABLE C: ARTICLE ANALYSIS SAMPLE

Study	Type of Study (Experimental / Quasi experimental / Controlled observational / Observ, no control groups / Expert opinion, consensus)	Research Methods	Population	Sample Size	Tools Used	Limitations	Major Findings	Criteria Guide
Giunta, F. and J. Rath (1969). "Effect of environmental illumination in prevention of hyperbilirubinemia of prematurity." Pediatrics 44(2): 162-7.	Experimental: x	Babies were randomly assigned to be either completely exposed in 90 footcandles or completely clothed in 10 footcandles for 6 days in the nursery. Eye shades were not used. All were in incubators.	Neonates were around 35 weeks gestational age, 45 males, mostly white. Neonates positive for Coomb's test were excluded.	96, 47 light group, 49 control group	Westinghouse light meter, Isolettes or Gordon Armstrong incubators, Evelyn-Malloy method for bilirubin detection, Coleman Junior Spectrophotometer	More work needs to be done on teasing apart the wavelength from the intensity. Higher light intensity has greater effects.	There were no significant differences on the first day, but by the last day there were highly significant differences. In the light treated group, only 3 babies developed indirect bilirubin levels over 15 mg, compared with 14 in the control group. Environmental lighting was effective in reducing bilirubin levels.	Good
Gold, K. J., D. W. Gorenflo, et al. (2006). "Physician experience with family presence during cardiopulmonary resuscitation in children." Pediatric Critical Care Medicine: A Journal of The Society of Critical Care Medicine and The World Federation of Pediatric Intensive and Critical Care Societies 7(5): 428-433.	Experimental: x	Providers were mailed a written survey that consisted of 40 multiple-choice and short-answer questions about demographics, past experiences and opinions on pediatric family presence.	Pediatric critical care and emergency medicine providers from professional association mailing lists; 99% of respondents were physicians.	521 surveys completed out of 1,200 surveys mailed	Survey and reminder cards; IRB approved	Conclusion was limited to 43% of physicians that did respond to survey and may or may not be applicable to the broader physician population that was surveyed.	The majority of respondents had resuscitated a child with family members present and thought that presence was helpful to parents and those residents should be trained in this practice. 93% of all respondents answered affirmatively when asked, "If you could make the decision, would you allow a family member to be present if they desired in at least some situations?" 68% of respondents reported that most parents wanted the option to be present. 74% believed family presence would be stressful for a resident physician.	Good
Gray, L. and M. Philbin (2005). "Effects of the neonatal intensive care unit on auditory attention and distraction." Clinical Perinatol 31: 243-260.	Expert opinion, consensus: x	Based on literature review about hearing science, the development of hearing, and noise environment in NICUs, the authors proposed a theory of auditory attention and distraction.	N/A	N/A	Literature review		Unpredictable background noise had detrimental effects on attention and distraction of listeners with different distractibility. Sound environments conducive to attention for an adult may detrimentally distract a child. Predictability of the acoustic environments, as well as relative loudness of the sound, was important for children's development. More attention should be paid to sound predictability in NICU.	Fair

APPENDIX | TABLE C: ARTICLE ANALYSIS SAMPLE | 79

Study	Type of Study: Experimental	Type of Study: Quasi experimental	Type of Study: Controlled observational	Type of Study: Observ., no control groups	Type of Study: Expert opinion, consensus	Research Methods	Population	Sample Size	Tools Used	Limitations	Major Findings	Criteria Guide
Griffin, T. (2003). "Facing challenges to family-centered care. I: Conflicts over visitation." Pediatric Nursing 29(2): 135-137.					x	Literature review and normative arguments	N/A	N/A	N/A	Normative arguments need support from evidence.	Family visitation can be a source of conflicts between families and nurses. To address this issue, flexible visitation guidelines (instead of rules) should be followed to meet families' needs. Nurses need to make adjustments to the policy change and help to increase family participation.	Fair
Griffin, T. (2003). "Facing challenges to family-centered care. II: Anger in the clinical setting." Pediatric Nursing 29(3): 212-214.					x	Literature review and normative arguments	N/A	N/A	N/A	Normative arguments need support from evidence.	Parental anger to nurses may result from: limited visitation, unexpected changes in patient health status, insufficient or conflicting information, and feeling ignored in patient care. To address this issue, nurses should apply the principals of family-centered care and develop strategies to handle these stressful situations.	Fair
Haiat, H., G. Bar-Mor, et al. (2003). "The world of the child: a world of play even in the hospital." Journal of Pediatric Nursing 18(3): 209-214.				x		The article described the integration of various aspects of game playing into the overall treatment approach at a pediatric hospital in Israel.	A pediatric hospital in Israel	1	Case study	Generalizability	Game play provided positive distractions. 2 projects were carried out to encourage play. 1 is a special playroom emulating a magical world. The other is a large playroom combining a computer area and an entertainment area. The new playrooms helped patients to better cope with the stress and better cooperate with treatments. Nurses should combine play with patient care to establish warm connection and trusting relationship.	Fair
Harris, D. D., M. M. Shepley, et al. (2006). "The impact of single family room design on patients and caregivers: executive summary." Journal of Perinatology 26: S38-S48			x			Literature review, plan reviews, site visits, post occupancy evaluations, construction cost analysis, evaluation of patient medical outcomes and surveys of health care staff	11 single family room, open-bay, combination and double-occupancy Level III NICUs in the United States	11	AutoCAD, construction cost data, anonymous aggregate personal health information, surveys	5 of the 11 hospital participants were able to provide hospital records.	Single family room care environments for NICUs provided solutions for increasing parent privacy and presence, supporting the Health Insurance Portability and Accountability Act compliance, minimizing the number of undesirable beds, increasing staff satisfaction and reducing staff stress.	Good

APPENDIX | TABLE C: ARTICLE ANALYSIS SAMPLE

Study	Type of Study (Experimental / Quasi experimental / Controlled observational / Observ., no control groups / Expert opinion, consensus)	Research Methods	Population	Sample Size	Tools Used	Limitations	Major Findings	Criteria Guide
Hofer, C., T. Abreu, et al. (2007). "Quality of hand hygiene in a pediatric hospital in Rio de Janerio, Brazil." Infect Control Hosp Epidemiol 28(5): 622-624.	Controlled observational (x)	A cross-sectional study of hand washing compliance by health care workers	Hand hygiene opportunities for all health care workers in a 60-bed tertiary pediatrics hospital	1,455	Covert observation	Probable confounding factors were not controlled.	Hang hygiene compliance rate was 34% (491 out of 1,455). Among these hand hygiene events, only 173 (35%) were performed correctly. Factors associated with correct performance of hand hygiene included: the use of alcohol-based products, a lack of jewelry and a higher nurse-to-patient ratio.	Fair
Holden, G., D. J. Bearison, et al. (2001). "The impact of a computer network on pediatric pain and anxiety: A randomized controlled clinical trial." Social Work in Health Care: The Journal of Health Care Social Work 36(2): 21-33.	Experimental (x)	Alternating treatment designs were administered randomly for a 30-minute period. Research assistant asked participants to rate their levels of pain intensity, pain aversiveness and anxiety.	Females and males between the ages 7-18; asthma was the predominant diagnosis in the sample.	39	Self report Visual Analog scale (VAS); Colored Analogue scale; Facial Affect scale; Anxiety scale	Technical problem with online program during a portion of the study	Children reported a high level of satisfaction with the implantation of the Starbright World (Starbright World-computer network intervention). Statistically significant results were observed in favor of SBW for pain intensity, pain adversiveness and anxiety. The effects appeared to be somewhat stronger for females and for children between the ages of 11 and 13.	Fair
Hutton, A. (2003). "Activities in the adolescent ward environment." Contemporary Nurse 14: 312-319.	Observ., no control groups (x)	Adolescent patients were asked to design their own ward and explain the reasons for the designs.	Adolescent patients (13-18 yr olds) who had chronic medical conditions and had frequent hospital admissions	7	Design drawing, interview	Small sample size, no comparison	Activity areas should be separated and away from other parts of the ward, provide spaces for a variety of activities and spaces for television.	Fair
Ispa, J., B. Barrett, et al. (1988). "Effects of Supervised Play in a Hospital Waiting Room." Children's Health Care 16(3): 195-200.	Quasi experimental (x)	Unobtrusive observations of patients and the accompanying adults were conducted in a waiting room. Supervised play was available during half of the observations (randomly selected) but not available in the other half of the observations.	Pediatric patients (5-10 year olds) and the accompanying adults in the waiting room of an outpatient clinic	30	Unobtrusive observation. Behavioral rating scales	Small sample size	Patients who were in the waiting room when supervised play was available were less anxious and cried less. Accompanying adults in the supervised play condition were less irritable and spoke with staff members more often.	Fair

APPENDIX | TABLE C: ARTICLE ANALYSIS SAMPLE | 81

Study	Type of Study (Experimental / Quasi experimental / Controlled observational / Observ, no control groups / Expert opinion, consensus)	Research Methods	Population	Sample Size	Tools Used	Limitations	Major Findings	Criteria Guide
Johnson, A. N. (2001). "Neonatal response to control of noise inside the incubator." Pediatric Nursing 27(6): 600-5.		Repeated measure, within subject, comparative design. Looked at sound levels, oxygen saturation and infant states in 3 conditions: pre-study in incubator, neonate with foam in incubator, post study without foam.	65 premature neonates. Mostly African American, 26-32 gestational weeks at birth	65	Quest model 2700, OB-100 Octave Filter Impulse Sound Level Meter with Sound Pressure Level; behavior measured using the Assessment of Preterm Infants' behavior; structured response observations with the Newborn Individualized Developmental Care and Assessment Program.	Generalizability	The use of foam decreased noise by an average of 3.27 decibels. The foam also had long term effects on the noise level. Not sure that the cost of the foam is balanced by the level of decrease.	Good
Judkins, S. (2003). "Paediatric emergency department design: Does it affect staff, patient and community satisfaction?" Emergency Medicine (Fremantle) 15(1): 63-7.	Observ, no control groups: x	Questionnaire surveys before and 6 months after the construction of a dedicated pediatric area in emergency department (ED)	Families of pediatric patients, general practitioners, ED staff member, and inpatient staff members in a Australia tertiary teaching hospital	93 family members, 148 general practitioners, 67 ED staff members and 38 inpatient staff members	Survey questionnaire	Small sample size on subgroups	Families were more satisfied with the physical environment and the overall care after the opening of the dedicated pediatric area. General practitioners referred more patients and were slightly more satisfied with the services. No improvements were found in the surveys of the ED and inpatient staff members.	Fair
Keipert, J. A. (1985). "The harmful effects of noise in a children's ward." Australian Paediatricians Journal 21(2): 101-3.	Observ, no control groups: x	Noise levels were measured and then interviews with staff were performed to find out about annoyance and effects of noise. The sound was examined in one of the 6-bed wards and was recorded for 12 minutes; there was another recorder at the nurses' station.	Registrars, resident medical officers, nursing sisters, medical social workers, play therapist in a children's ward	2, 2, 4, 2 and 1 (respectively), 11 total	General Radio 1982 sound level meter and analyzer, used on the A scale because similar to what the human ear picks up. Interviews were also conducted.	No statistical or qualitative analysis of the interviews; no means for the noise levels; only taken during one 12-minute period (not generalizable); recordings only took place in one area.	All those who were interviewed thought the noise was excessive, interfered with work ability and effects of noise were worse when pressure at work was high. Next to the cleaning machines, the crying of infants was very annoying. Other bothersome noises were running, yelling, noisy toys, telephones, etc. The noise levels during the 12 minutes ranged from 52 (rare) to 90.	Fair

APPENDIX | TABLE C: ARTICLE ANALYSIS SAMPLE

Study	Type of Study (Experimental / Quasi experimental / Controlled observational / Observ., no control groups / Expert opinion, consensus)	Research Methods	Population	Sample Size	Tools Used	Limitations	Major Findings	Criteria Guide
Kent, W. D., A. K. Tan, et al. (2002). "Excessive noise levels in the neonatal ICU: Potential effects on auditory system development." Journal of Otolaryngology 31(6).	Observ., no control groups: x	Looked at noise in 2 phases: 1) staff activity and 2) ambient noise. Recordings occurred over a 6-day period with 12-hour recoding sessions (this was for Phase 1). Phase 2 had recording for 4 days and 24 hours a day.	NICU comprised of 4 rooms each with 6 patients, 1 acute patient room	1 NICU, 4 rooms	Sound level meter (model 712 Larson Davis, Provo, UT) with 3/8 in pre-polarized microphone (model 2541, Larson Davis)-used an A filter	No manipulation of staff activity, no manipulation of the environmental factors	The rooms had significantly higher noise levels than recommended. Staff is a major contributor to the noise levels.	Good
Larson, E, S Albrecht, and Mary O'Keefe. 2005. Hand hygiene behavior in a pediatric emergency department and a pediatric intensive care unit: Comparison of use of 2 dispenser systems. American Journal of Critical Care 14 (4): 304-11.	Quasi experimental: x	The usage of 2 types of dispensers of alcohol sanitizer (manual and hands-free) was compared. Counting devices were used to record the usage. Each type of dispenser was placed for one 2-month period in a pediatric emergency department and a PICU. To control for an order effect, a crossover design was used. In addition, hand hygiene compliance was recorded by observation.	Alcohol sanitizers, indications for hand hygiene	37 alcohol sanitizers, 5,568 indications for hand hygiene	Counting devices, observation	The usage of hands-free sanitizer might not be accurately counted because the sanitizer might dispense even when staff inadvertently entered the sensor zone without hand hygiene.	The touch-free sanitizers were used significantly more often than the manual sanitizers. The overall hand hygiene compliance rate was 38.4% and did not differ between the emergency department and the PICU.	Fair

APPENDIX | TABLE C: ARTICLE ANALYSIS SAMPLE | 83

Study	Type of Study					Research Methods	Population	Sample Size	Tools Used	Limitations	Major Findings	Criteria Guide
	Experimental	Quasi experimental	Controlled observational	Observ., no control groups	Expert opinion, consensus							
Larson, E. L., J. Cimiotti, et al. (2005). "Effect of antiseptic hand washing vs. alcohol sanitizer on health care-associated infections in neonatal intensive care units." Archives of Pediatrics & Adolescent Medicine 159(4): 377-383.		x				Each hand hygiene product was used for 11 consecutive months; surveillance was conducted by a nurse epidemiologist who visited the units 3 times per week, collected neonatal data, performed monthly noninvasive assessments of nurses' skin conditions, observer assessment to examine hands, self assessment of skin condition, microbial counts on nurses' hands and nurses recorded a diary 1 shift per month.	43-bed unit NICU I and 50-bed NICU II; full time nurses and all neonates hospitalized for more than 24 hours were eligible for inclusion.	2,932 neonatal hospital admissions and 119 nurse participants	Hand hygiene products, noninvasive assessment tools to assess nurses' skin condition, modified glove juice technique, self-assessment	Multiple contributory factors including patient risk, unit design and staff behavior	Infection rates and microbial counts on nurses' hands were equivalent during hand washing and alcohol phases. Nurses skin condition was improved using alcohol. Systems-level interventions are needed to improve the quality of hand hygiene practices.	Good
Levy, G. D., D. J. Woolston, et al. (2003). "Mean noise amounts in Level II vs. Level III neonatal intensive care units." Neonatal Network 22(2): 33-39.				x		Group design measurements were taken near the center of each NICU. Decibel amounts were recorded every 30 seconds for about 25 minutes at a time. They were between 11 and 1,125, and 4 and 425.	Five Level II NICUs and 7 Level III NICUs	12, 5 and 7	A Quest 215 Type II Sound Level Meter with A scale filter	There is no analysis for what is causing the noise.	Controlled for number of infants in the ward. Found that there was significantly greater noise in Level III than Level II. Greatest noise for most medically fragile infants.	Good
Lewis, M., M. Bendersky, et al. (1991). "Visitation to a neonatal intensive care unit." Pediatrics 88(4): 795-800.				x		Visiting logs, medical records and interviews with mothers of preterm newborns were examined to determine which factors contribute to the variation in visitation.	Mothers of preterm newborns in a NICU	164	Visiting logs recorded by nurses, medical records, Hollingshead Four-Factor Index of parental educational and occupational level	Correlational study	Newborns had more days with no visitors if they had intraventricular hemorrhages, their parents did not live together with them and they were not firstborn. If the mother was hospitalized, her condition was the only contributing factor. The worse the mother's condition, the more likely the newborn had no visitors.	Fair

84 | **APPENDIX** | **TABLE C: ARTICLE ANALYSIS SAMPLE**

Study	Type of Study (Experimental / Quasi experimental / Controlled observational / Observ., no control groups / Expert opinion, consensus)	Research Methods	Population	Sample Size	Tools Used	Limitations	Major Findings	Criteria Guide
Loewy, J., C. Hallan, et al. (2005). "Sleep/sedation in children undergoing EEG testing: a comparison of chloral hydrate and music therapy." Journal of PeriAnesthesia Nursing 20(5): 323-332.	Quasi experimental: x	Based on day of week admitted, patients were either assigned to the Chloral Hydrate (CH) or music therapy (MT) group. 30 minutes were allotted to allow the intervention to be successful; if it was not after 30 minutes, the other intervention would be employed. In the CH group, patients received 60 mg/kg of the sedative orally, the music was chosen by the caregiver. Subjects were sleep deprived and could not eat close to surgery. Data collected before, during and after surgery. 7 music therapists used.	1 month to 5 years, inpatients all going through EEGs	60	Chloral Hydrate, live music therapy, the Beth Israel Medical Center flow sheet sedation scale		In the music therapy group, only 2.9% needed the additional intervention, in the sedation group, 50% needed the additional intervention. This was significant. The mean time to fall sleep in the CH group was 32 minutes, compared with 23 minutes in the music group, but not significant. The length of sleep was significantly shorter in the MT group. Level of sleep was also significant (lower for music).	Good
Macnab, A., P. Thiessen, et al. (2000). "Parent assessment of family-centered care practices in a children's hospital." Children's Health Care 29(2): 113-128.	Observ., no control groups: x	Telephone interview survey of parents three to four weeks after discharge for their opinions of family centered care	Parents of acute pediatric patients in a tertiary children's hospital	39	Clinical Consumer Survey - a telephone questionnaire survey with 125 structured and open-ended questions	Descriptive, no comparisons	Parents were willing to provide feedback to improve family centered care. Overall, the interviewed parents were satisfied with the care. But study identified several areas to be improved. About 49% of parents felt angry on some issues of care. Over 40% of parents reported contradictions in the answers provided by physicians and nurses.	Fair

APPENDIX | TABLE C: ARTICLE ANALYSIS SAMPLE | 85

Study	Type of Study: Experimental	Type of Study: Quasi experimental	Type of Study: Controlled observational	Type of Study: Observ., no control groups	Type of Study: Expert opinion, consensus	Research Methods	Population	Sample Size	Tools Used	Limitations	Major Findings	Criteria Guide
McDonald, L. C., M. Walker, et al. (1998). "Outbreak of Acinetobacter spp. bloodstream infections in a nursery associated with contaminated aerosols and air conditioners." The Pediatric Infectious Disease Journal 17(8): 716-22.			x			A retrospective cohort study was conducted in a special care nursery after an outbreak of Acinetobacter spp. Environmental cultures and air samples were tested for contamination.	Patients in a special care nursery during the outbreak period	33	Laboratory test, air sampling, environmental cultures	Air conditioners were only one of several possible routes of infection transmission that the study suggested.	Patients with peripheral IV catheters were more likely to be infected. Contact with one specific nurse was an independent risk factor for infection, suggesting that hand contact might play a role in transmission. Cultures from the ventilation grates and external surface of air conditioners were positive for A. lwoffii. Air conditioners might be important in pathogen transmission.	Fair
Moore, K. A. C., K. Coker, et al. (2003). "Implementing potentially better practices for improving family-centered care in neonatal intensive care units: Successes and challenges." Pediatrics 111(4): e450-e460.				x		Case studies of 11 NICUs' collaboration in improving family centered care	Medical centers participating in a NICU quality improvement collaboration	11	Potentially better practice areas were identified through a process of self-analysis, review of literature, site visits, expert consultation. Improvements were made and evaluated in the potentially better practice areas.	Limited comparisons, qualitative	Family centered care is more of a process than a destination. Different NICUs were at different stages in supporting family centered care. Full family participation requires family's unlimited access to the units, which could result in higher satisfaction.	Fair
Morrison, W. E., E. Haas, et al. (2003). "Noise, stress, and annoyance in a pediatric intensive care unit." Critical Care Medicine 31(1): 113-119.			x			During a 3-hour period of patient care, each nurse's heart rate and environmental sound level were recorded continuously; saliva samples and stress ratings were recorded every 30 minutes. Multiple regression analysis was used to detect predictors of stress.	Registered nurses in a PICU in a tertiary care hospital	11	Audiogram, salivary amylase, Holter monitor, Pediatric Risk of Mortality Score, The Specific Rating of Events Scale by the US Army Research Laboratory stress program	Small sample size	Higher average sound level was a significant predictor of higher heart rate, higher subjective stress and annoyance. Other predictors of higher heart rate included higher caffeine intake, less nursing experience and daytime shift. Amylase measurements were not predicted by noise level.	Fair

APPENDIX | TABLE C: ARTICLE ANALYSIS SAMPLE

Study	Type of Study (Experimental / Quasi experimental / Controlled observational / Observ., no control groups / Expert opinion, consensus)	Research Methods	Population	Sample Size	Tools Used	Limitations	Major Findings	Criteria Guide
Mulhall, A., D. Kelly, et al. (2004). "A qualitative evaluation of an adolescent cancer unit." European Journal of Cancer Care 13: 16-22.	Observ., no control groups (x)	The study utilized observation and interview to qualitatively evaluate the first adolescent oncology unit in the UK.	Pediatric patients, parents, staff members	10 patients, 10 parents, 14 staff members	Observation, interview	Small sample size	Adolescent cancer patients have special care and treatment needs. Physical environment was 1 of the 6 themes emerged from the data. Positive distractions, such as day room, pool table and music, helped to promote a feeling of normality. Staff members reported the lack of space and privacy in the unit. However patients reported the smallness provided a sense of intimacy.	Fair
Pass, M. and R. Bolig (1993). "A comparison of play behaviors in two child life program variations." Child Health Care. 22(1): 5-17.	Controlled observational (x)	Unobtrusive observations of preschool patient play behaviors in playrooms	Pre-school patients in 4 units of a pediatric hospital and the pediatric unit of a general hospital	15	Observation	Small sample size. No control on various confounding variables	More non-play behaviors (e.g. conversation, transition between activities, eating and feeding fish) were exhibited in playroom-focused setting (group) than in non-playroom-focused setting (individual). No differences in play behaviors were found. Gender, length of stay and disease type contributed to significant differences in play behaviors.	Fair
Pati, D. and P. Barach (In Review). "Impact of View on Nurse Well Being: An Exploratory Study on Chronic Stress, Acute Stress and Alertness."	Observ., no control groups (x)	Multiple regression analysis on the relationship between the duration of exterior view and the stress level of nurses. Questionnaire survey was used to collected data. The effect of view content was suggested.	32 registered nurses from 19 units of 2 children's hospitals	32	Questionnaire survey, Perceived Stress Scale, Stress/Arousal Adjective Checklist, Revised Nursing Work Index	Small sample size. The result of regression analysis (positive relation between view and stress) was contradicted with subsequent descriptive analysis of data from subgroups.	Multiple regression analysis showed positive relation between view duration and arousal/stress. But subsequent descriptive analysis of subgroups suggested a beneficial effect of view duration on stress. The data suggested that nature view over non-nature view had a beneficial impact on nurse stress.	Fair

APPENDIX | TABLE C: ARTICLE ANALYSIS SAMPLE | 87

Study	Type of Study (Experimental / Quasi experimental / Controlled observational / Observ., no control groups / Expert opinion, consensus)	Research Methods	Population	Sample Size	Tools Used	Limitations	Major Findings	Criteria Guide
Pati, D. and T. Harvey (In Review). "Taking Care of Our Nurses."	Observ., no control groups (x)	The study looked at 3 questions: do views of nature effect chronic stress, acute stress, response readiness? Prior to and following the shift, nurses from 19 unit types were asked questions regarding to stress levels. Other factors that could affect stress were also accounted for.	Nurses from 19 unit types	More than 30	Survey	The study does not have specific numbers, no listing of the limitations, brief analyses	Views of nature can affect acute stress, but were not as effective at affecting chronic stress. Furthermore, readiness was higher for nurses with views of nature.	Good
Pelander, T. and H. Leino-Kilpi (2004). "Quality in pediatric nursing care: children's expectations." Issues Comprehensive Pediatric Nursing 27(3): 139-151.	Observ., no control groups (x)	Theme interviews conducted based on literature review of topic. The thematic entities covered children's expectations related to nurses, nursing activities and environment.	Children of preschool and school age either with chronic diseases or hospitalized for a short period were recruited to the study	20 pre-school-aged children and 20 school-age children	Interviews within patient rooms or examination rooms		The purpose of this study was to describe children's expectations concerning the quality of nursing care. The characteristics expected from the nurse were humanity, a sense of humor and reliability. The children expected the nurses to be cheerful, funny, amusing. They also expected entertainment from nurses.	Fair
Perkins, A. M. and J. R. Buchhalter (2006). "Optimizing patient care in the pediatric epilepsy monitoring unit." Journal of Neuroscience Nursing 38(6): 416.	Observ., no control groups (x)	Multidisciplinary discussions and surveys of nurses working in a pediatric epilepsy monitoring unit (PEMU) to identify areas of nursing confidence. Findings allowed hospital to refine aspects of patient care and implement an educational program for nurses who work in the PEMU; survey (IRB approved) was implemented to further determine nurses' perceptions related to the implementation of interventions and their comfort level working in the PEMU.	Nurses who worked in the PEMU participated in survey; feedback from parents and patients was also recorded.	37 out of 84 surveyed responded	Survey		Suggestions included providing education before admission to family, seizure precautions instituted in patient rooms, install white boards for feedback in patient rooms, develop PEMU checklist for staff reference, standardize medication administration order set, identify RNs to serve as clinical leaders. Careful attention to detail in the areas of unit design, nurse education, family expectations and education, medication administration and communication was suggested.	Fair

APPENDIX | TABLE C: ARTICLE ANALYSIS SAMPLE

Study	Type of Study (Experimental / Quasi experimental / Controlled observational / Observ., no control groups / Expert opinion, consensus)	Research Methods	Population	Sample Size	Tools Used	Limitations	Major Findings	Criteria Guide
Polkki, T., K. Vehvilainen, et al. (2001). "Nonpharmacological methods in relieving children's postoperative pain: a survey on hospital nurses in Finland." Journal of Advanced Nursing 34(2): 483-492.	Observ., no control groups: x	Descriptive study, 8 wards, 5 hospitals	Finish nurses of 8-12 yr olds patients	162	Questionnaire		Used many factors often: television/video, books (distraction), environment changes (noise, belongings); sometimes: books (prep), demos, fames, music, crafts, temperature, interior design.	Good
Rassin, M., Y. Gutman, et al. (2004). "Developing a Computer Game to Prepare Children for Surgery." Association of Perioperative Registered Nurses 80(6): 1095-1196.	Observ., no control groups: x	Literature review of the use of computer game in preparing children for surgery and interviews with sick and healthy children regarding games	Children awaiting surgery and healthy children	10 children awaiting surgery, 10 healthy children	Content analysis	Small sample size. No description about the genders of respondents	Children reported anesthetization and pain as main source of fears and concerns. Most children were not interested in information about surgery. Children preferred interactive games with an adventure scenario, cartoon characters and competitive elements.	Fair
Rice, B. A. and C. Nelson (2005). "Safety in the Pediatric ICU: The Key to Quality Outcomes." Critical Care Nursing Clinics of North America 17(4): 431-440.	Expert opinion, consensus: x	Literature review and normative argument	N/A	N/A	N/A	Normative arguments need support from evidence.	To improve patient safety, PICUs should standardize care processes, use redundancy and maintain transparency. Major issues in patient safety included: effective communications, mortality prediction, severity of illness adjusted length of stay, patient identification, catheter-related bloodstream infections, unplanned endotracheal extubations, restraints and medication safety.	Fair

APPENDIX | TABLE C: ARTICLE ANALYSIS SAMPLE | 89

Study	Type of Study					Research Methods	Population	Sample Size	Tools Used	Limitations	Major Findings	Criteria Guide
	Experimental	Quasi experimental	Controlled observational	Observ., no control groups	Expert opinion, consensus							
Robb, S. L. (2000). "The effect of therapeutic music interventions on the behavior of hospitalized children in isolation: Developing a contextual support model of music therapy." Journal of Music Therapy 37(2): 118-146.	x					Pediatric patients were videotaped in four 15-minute sessions in their own private rooms. The first and last sessions served as controls, including normal hospital activities, such as TV, play and brief medical procedures. In the second session, patients read the book with a therapist when listening to a sound recording of a storybook. In the third session, patients listened to music with the therapist. Patient mood was recorded during each session. The videotaping was later analyzed.	Pediatric oncology patients restricted to an isolated environment	10	Videotaping, Affective Face Scale	Small sample size. Low generalizability	Patients received more support from adults and elicited more engaging behaviors in music therapy condition than in other conditions. No significant difference was found in mood scores in all conditions.	Fair
Said, I. (2003). Design Consideration and Construction Process of Children Therapeutic Garden. International Conference on Construction Technology: 15.				x		Questionnaires and interviews of pediatric patients and their caregivers regarding patients' interactions with gardens	Patients or their caregivers in the pediatric wards of 2 hospitals in Malaysia	360	Questionnaire/survey	Limited description of the study. The major part of the article is a description of the design process.	Patient's interactions with garden contributed to better psychological status. Most patients preferred staying and playing in the garden. Beneficial garden features included refreshing scent, fresh air, ample light, view, home feeling and variety of places for activities.	Poor
Said, I., S. S. Salleh, et al. (2005). "Caregivers' Evaluation on Hospitalized Children's Preferences Concerning Garden and Ward." Journal of Asian Architecture and Building Engineering 4(2): 331-338.				x		Questionnaire surveys were conducted to evaluate pediatric patients' usage of and behavioral responses to gardens beside the pediatric wards.	The mothers of patients and the nurses in the pediatric wards of 2 hospitals in Malaysia	360 mothers, 43 nurses	Questionnaire/survey	Minimal comparison, descriptive analysis	The mothers reported that their children preferred staying in gardens than in wards. The gardens were rated higher than the wards in the following features: refreshing smell, fresh air, ample light, cheerful, pleasant sound, scenic view, open space, free to play, home feeling, not confined and variety of places for activities. Nurses evaluated the gardens as beneficial. The behaviors of patients changed positively.	Fair

APPENDIX | **TABLE C: ARTICLE ANALYSIS SAMPLE**

Study	Type of Study: Experimental	Quasi experimental	Controlled observational	Observ., no control groups	Expert opinion, consensus	Research Methods	Population	Sample Size	Tools Used	Limitations	Major Findings	Criteria Guide
Saunders, A. N. (1995). "Incubator noise: a method to decrease decibels." Pediatric Nursing 21(3): 265-8.			x			Noise level measurements were taken to measure noise outside the incubators, inside the uncovered incubators and inside covered incubators of premature infants during 2 random days each week over a 3-week period in the fall of 1993.	Premature infants	24	Sound level meter to measure decibel levels		Data from this study shows covering the incubator decreases noise for the infant inside under all conditions. There was a difference in all noise levels between inside and outside measurements. In every case, incubator noise levels decreased with the application of covering. Research is ongoing to establish standards for noise levels in infant environments. The developmental impact of hearing loss is well documented in research; the significant results of this study strongly suggest the necessity for these interventions and call for additional research on methods of noise control inside the incubator.	Good
Saunders, R. P., M. R. Abraham, et al. (2003). "Evaluation and development of potentially better practices for improving family-centered care in neonatal intensive care units." Pediatrics 111(4): e437-e449.			x			The collaboration process of improving family centered care was implemented. It included: internal process analysis, literature review, focus group, benchmark site visits to NICUs of excellence in family centered care. Questionnaire survey tools were developed to measure parent-reported outcomes, and care provider's beliefs and practices. Clinical outcomes were compared, including length of stay, feeding and incidence of chronic lung disease.	NICUs of 11 medical centers, parents and staff members	11	Questionnaire/survey		No differences were found in clinical outcomes before (1998) and after (2000) the collaboration process. Survey questionnaires to measure parental outcomes and staff beliefs and practices were developed.	Fair

APPENDIX | TABLE C: ARTICLE ANALYSIS SAMPLE | 91

Study	Type of Study					Research Methods	Population	Sample Size	Tools Used	Limitations	Major Findings	Criteria Guide
	Experimental	Quasi experimental	Controlled observational	Observ., no control groups	Expert opinion, consensus							
Shepley, M. (2002). "Predesign and postoccupancy analysis of staff behavior in a neonatal intensive care unit." Children's Health Care 31(3): 237-253.				x		Literature review	N/A	N/A	Literature review		Design interventions that provided positive distraction and can be introduced into the NICU setting were window views of pleasant outside vistas, soothing artwork and the ability to listen to music.	Good
Shepley, M. (2006). "The role of positive distraction in neonatal intensive care unit settings." Journal of Perinatology 26: S34-S37.				x		Multi-methodological approach: Pre-design research and post occupancy evaluation, which included behavioral mapping, interviews, questionnaires and calibrated measures of walking, noise and temperature.	NICU	1 original unit NICU and the new unit contrasting in efficiency of plan configuration (multi-room vs. open plan), total area and provision of family centered care.	Questionnaires, behavioral mapping and interviews		Total amount of time staff spent walking from activity to activity was not reduced when infant beds were distributed in an open floor plan with 60% more area, however when the data was weighted to reflect the impact of the size of the unit, the ratio of time spent traveling to a total unit area was found to be less in the open-bay plan.	Good
Sherman, S. A., J. W. Varni, et al. (2005). "Post-occupancy evaluation of healing gardens in a pediatric cancer center." Landscape and Urban Planning 73(2-3): 167-183.				x		Post occupancy evaluation; demographic information, activities and length of stay were recorded; behavioral observations, window use observation	Pediatric cancer center garden users	1,400; Pilot data: 22	Pediatric Quality of Life Inventory	Pilot data: sample size small	The majority of visitors were adults who mostly engaged in sedentary activities. Children who used the garden interacted with garden features significantly more than adults. Emotional distress and pain are lower for all groups when in the gardens than when inside the hospital.	Good
Sherman, S., M. Shepley, et al. (2005). "Children's environments and health-related quality of life: evidence informing pediatric healthcare environmental design." Children, Youth and Environments 15(1): 188-223.					x	Literature review and theorization	Literature on the effects of children's environments (including health care) on health-related quality of life	40 studies	Literature search and review		Access to nature, lower noise level, reduced crowding, music and soft lighting that promotes circadian rhythms, were related to better outcomes.	Good

APPENDIX | TABLE C: ARTICLE ANALYSIS SAMPLE

Study	Type of Study (Experimental / Quasi experimental / Controlled observational / Observ., no control groups / Expert opinion, consensus)	Research Methods	Population	Sample Size	Tools Used	Limitations	Major Findings	Criteria Guide
Smith, A., G. Hefley, et al. (2007). "Parent Bed Spaces in the PICU: Effect on Parental Stress." Pediatric Nursing.	Controlled observational: x	Parental Stressor Scale, demographic questionnaire, taken of parental groups before and after 2 hospitals created bed spaces for parents	Parents from 2 free standing tertiary care children's hospitals in south central U.S. Parents, guardians, stepparents of children who have spent at least 2 nights in the hospital	138 mothers, 34 fathers, 2 guardians, 3 stepparents	Scale (with tested validity and reliability) and questionnaire		Parental stress significantly decreased in the new facilities with parental bed spaces. The confounding variable was that in addition to bed spaces, the parents were also no longer confined to specific visiting hours and could stay with their children 24 hrs a day. There were also difference between ethnic groups and this might require more extensive study.	Good
Thear, G. and R. A. Wittmann-Price (2006). "Project noise buster in the NICU: how one facility lowered noise levels when caring for preterm infants." American Journal of Nursing 106(5): 64AA.	Controlled observational: x	Data was collected before and after interventions. A decimeter at six zones in the NICU was used. Staff was informed of the data collection but not of the nature of the study. The interventions used were noise indicator lights that signaled when noise was above 60 db, an hour of quiet time at 3 different times, changes in nursing care schedule, verbal instruction to parents about noise, memo about new protocol to ancillary people, structural changes—double doors were replaced with quieter doors.	In the NICU, but there was no study on actual patients, just noise levels.	NA	Decimeter in 6 zones	Staff knew data was being collected, a number of changes were done at once, so difficult to extrapolate which changes really made the difference. There was not data collection for culture change.	Noise levels were lower in all 6 zones; the greatest decrease was near the new doors. Even after 3, 6 and 12 months, the noise was still lowered. Culture in the unit also changed.	Fair

APPENDIX | TABLE C: ARTICLE ANALYSIS SAMPLE | 93

Study	Type of Study					Research Methods	Population	Sample Size	Tools Used	Limitations	Major Findings	Criteria Guide
	Experimental	Quasi experimental	Controlled observational	Observ., no control groups	Expert opinion, consensus							
Van Blerkom, L. M. (1995). "Clown Doctors: Shaman Healers of Western Medicine." Medical Anthropology Quarterly 9(4): 14.				x		Participant-observation of a critical care unit (CCU) clown doctors. Written record was kept of time, context, actors, clowns' actions and patient/nurse reactions. The clown's behavior was the main observational focus. Interviews were conducted with CCU clowns. A literature review comparing western medical practices and non-western therapies along with comparing shamans with clowns. Written evaluations of the CCU from parents and hospital staff were utilized.	5 groups of clown doctors	Undetermined	Participant observation, written evaluation, meeting presence and literature review		The clown helped the patient and family provide meaning to the illness experience and resolve personal and social problems that resulted from it which in turn increased patient satisfaction, compliance and perhaps outcome.	Poor
Varni, J. W., T. M. Burwinkle, et al. (2004). "Evaluation of the built environment at a Children's Convalescent Hospital: Development of the Pediatric Quality of Life Inventory (TM) parent and staff satisfaction measures for pediatric health care facilities." Journal of Developmental and Behavioral Pediatrics 25(1): 10-20.				x		Focus groups were conducted to develop the Pediatric Quality of Life Inventory measuring parent and staff satisfaction with physical environment, health care services and coworker relationship in a pediatric skilled nursing facility. The measurement instruments were tested in a mail survey.	Parents of pediatric patients with chronic medical conditions, staff members	40 parents, 72 staff members	Pediatric Quality of Life Inventory	Generalizability. Small sample size for factor analysis	The measurement instruments demonstrated internal consistency reliability and initial construct validity. Parent satisfaction with physical environment was positively associated with parent satisfaction with health care services. Staff satisfaction with physical environment was positively associated with staff satisfaction with coworker relationship.	Good

APPENDIX | TABLE C: ARTICLE ANALYSIS SAMPLE

Study	Type of Study (Experimental / Quasi experimental / Controlled observational / Observ., no control groups / Expert opinion, consensus)	Research Methods	Population	Sample Size	Tools Used	Limitations	Major Findings	Criteria Guide
Walsh, W. F., K. L. McCullough, et al. (2006). "Room for improvement: nurses' perceptions of providing care in a single room newborn intensive care setting." Advances in Neonatal Care 6(5): 261-270.	Controlled observational: x	Questionnaire survey of nurses' perceptions of new single room NICU compared to the old open unit. Sound level and infection rate in the new NICU were measured and compared with the old open unit.	NICU nurses	127	Questionnaire survey, sound level meter	One-time survey. No before-after comparison	Nurses reported that single rooms were better in quality of patient care, hand washing and parent satisfaction. However, there were challenges due to single rooms, including insufficient staffing, lower visibility, more difficult monitoring and longer walking distance because of the larger unit. Both noise level and infection rate were significantly lower in the new single room unit.	Fair
Walworth, D. D. (2005). "Procedural-support music therapy in the healthcare setting: a cost-effectiveness analysis." Journal of Pediatric Nursing 20(4): 276-284.	Observ., no control groups: x	Patients undergoing ECGs and other procedures to look at when patients did not need sedation because they had the music therapy. In the waiting area before the procedure, patients were asked what kind of music they preferred.	The patients were pediatric patients in a general medical hospital receiving ECG (92), CT scans (57) or other procedures (17)	166	The tools were live music (including guitar, rhythm instruments and visual aids). The only tool to evaluate effectiveness was whether or not the patient fell asleep for the procedure.	There were no tools evaluating the method, the feelings of the patients or how the caregivers felt about the procedure. Purely observation. Furthermore, the patients might have been solely reacting to the fact that they had an additional person soothing them. No way to tease that from the live music.	100% of ECG patients, 80.7% of CT patients, and 94.1% other procedure patients were able to fall asleep without any sedation - just the assistance of live music. Other analyses (not identified) show that music therapy saves money, time and resources.	Good
White, R. (2003). "Individual Rooms in the NICU- an evolving concept." Journal of Perinatology 23(Supplement 1): S22-S24.	Expert opinion, consensus: x	The article discussed the advantages and disadvantages of single rooms in NICU and proposed suggestions for design.	N/A	N/A	N/A	Only 4 references were listed.	The advantages of single rooms in NICU included individualized environmental stimuli, privacy and family presence. The disadvantages included difficulty for nursing staff in patient care, the isolation of families, and extra cost and space demands. To overcome the disadvantages, rooms should be clustered in groups of 6 or more and electronic devices can be used for communication.	Fair

APPENDIX | TABLE C: ARTICLE ANALYSIS SAMPLE | 95

Study	Type of Study: Experimental / Quasi experimental / Controlled observational / Observ, no control groups / Expert opinion, consensus	Research Methods	Population	Sample Size	Tools Used	Limitations	Major Findings	Criteria Guide
Wolitzky, K., R. Fivush, et al. (2005). "Effectiveness of virtual reality distraction during a painful medical procedure in pediatric oncology patients." Psychology & Health 20(6): 817-824.		Pediatric oncology patients were randomly assigned to either receive virtual reality (VR) or no VR. The patients were asked to fill out information on how they feel. After the procedure, patients were asked to give a narrative about what happened during their visit to the hospital. Patients were given movie tickets as a thank you for participating.	Aged 7-14 yr olds, oncology patients, undergoing a port access procedure in a major metropolitan city	23	VR system for children visiting the gorilla exhibit at the zoo, How-I-Feel questionnaire, pulse, Visual Analogue Scale for pain and anxiety, The Children's Hospital of Eastern Ontario Pain Scale	There was a lot of variation in age and number/type of previous procedures, small sample, only one coder, needed to have looked at mediators of distress.	There was a significant decrease in stress and pain for the VR group. There were no significant differences going into the procedure. Patients in the VR group also remembered significantly more narrative details than the control group.	Good

3 | THE BUSINESS CASE FOR BUILDING BETTER PEDIATRIC FACILITIES

Business Case

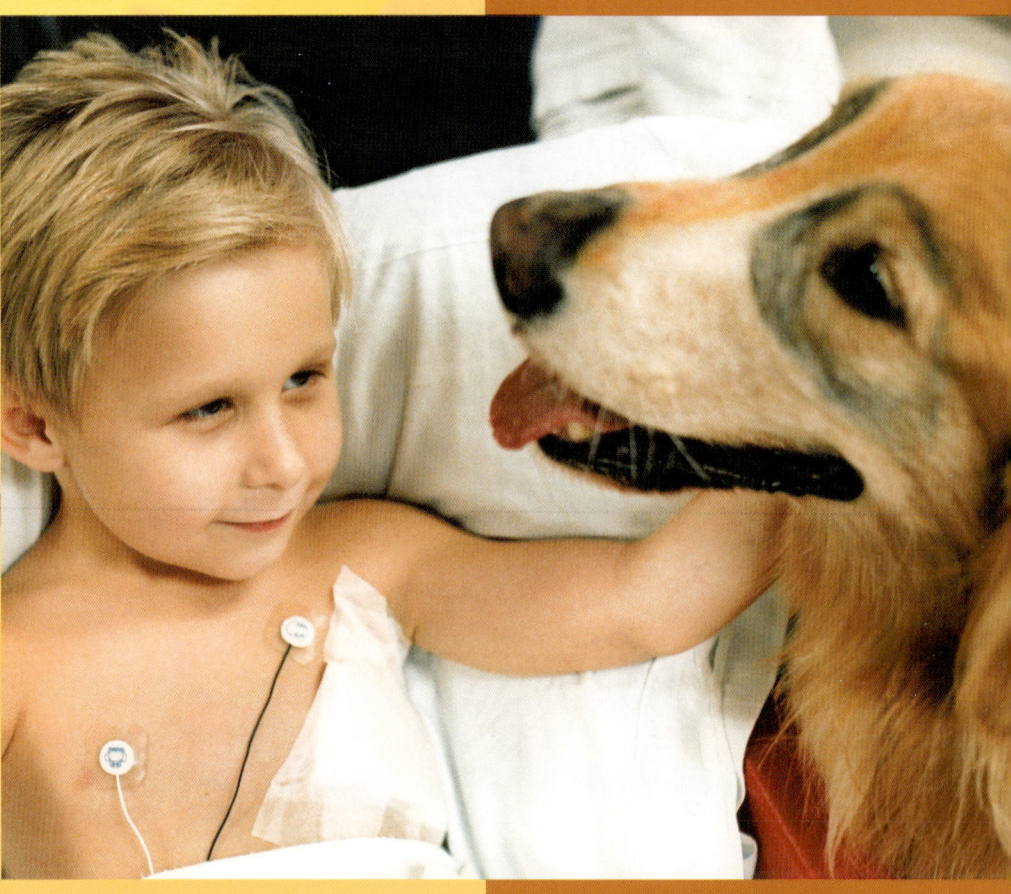

No tricks here — just treats as a pet therapy dog makes a boy's Halloween in the hospital special. Photo by Jennifer T. Foley, Arnold Palmer Hospital for Children & Women Orlando Regional Healthcare System, Orlando, FL

BLAIR L. SADLER, J.D.
Past President and Chief Executive Officer
Rady Children's Hospital, San Diego
Senior Fellow, Institute for Healthcare Improvement

JENNIFER R. DUBOSE, M.S., LEED AP
Research Associate II
Georgia Institute of Technology

CRAIG ZIMRING, Ph.D.
Professor of Architecture and Psychology
Georgia Institute of Technology

> We shape our buildings;
> thereafter they shape us.
> —Winston Churchill

For decades, the nation's children's hospitals have been leaders in providing state-of-the-art patient care, undertaking important breakthroughs in basic and translation research, teaching the next generation of pediatric doctors and nurses, and informing communities about the importance of child health care issues through effective advocacy. Children's hospitals have also been leaders in providing positive healing environments through programs (art therapy), policies (open ended visiting hours) and buildings where care is provided (larger single patient rooms where a family member can stay overnight with a child). Today, many children's hospitals are undertaking major construction projects while others are considering important upgrades to existing facilities. NACHRI estimates that there are 250-275 children's hospitals in the United States. Of these, 50-55 are freestanding acute care children's hospitals; 110-125 are acute care children's hospitals within larger hospitals; and 90-100 are orthopedic, rehabilitative, psychiatric and other specialty children's hospitals.

Just as in adult health care systems, pediatric hospitals and their leaders are confronting numerous challenging and often competing demands: unpredictable reimbursement, workforce shortages, skyrocketing costs, increasing disclosure requirements, mounting consumer and employer expectations and aggressive union tactics. Most relevant, a patient quality and safety revolution is sweeping the country (Institute of Medicine, 2000, 2001). Consumers, employers and payers are demanding that hospitals dramatically reduce system-based errors, which harm, even kill thousands of patients annually (Sadler, 2006b).

The speed of the quality revolution has accelerated dramatically, spurred on by converging forces, including: the Leapfrog Group[1] on behalf of employers; pay-for-performance or value-based purchasing efforts, such as the Centers for Medicare and Medicaid Services (CMS)/Premier Hospital Quality Incentive Demonstration project[2], which are being adopted in various forms by individual states and commercial payers; greater emphasis by The Joint Commission in its standards to improve safety and quality[3]; as well as two innovative nationwide campaigns coordinated by the Institute for Healthcare Improvement (IHI)[4]. The IHI 100,000 Lives Campaign was sufficiently successful in helping to reduce deaths to patients; so in late 2006, IHI led the design and announcement of a second campaign, Protecting 5 Million Lives from Harm, which includes 12 specific areas of intervention. A Pediatric Affinity Group, led by the National Initiative for Children's Healthcare Quality (NICHQ), National Association of Children's Hospitals and Related Institutions (NACHRI), Child Health Corporation of America (CHCA), American Academy of Pediatrics and several mentor hospitals, formed to adjust certain of the interventions for children's health care. The Institute for Family Centered Care has actively supported the initiative. Over 3,700 hospitals are now participating in this campaign (Institute for Healthcare Improvement, 2008). In addition to clinicians and managers, hospital boards of trustees are now being encouraged to get much more involved.

At the same time, many hospital facilities, including children's hospitals, have simply come to the end of their useful lives, and in several states, seismic requirements are mandating major facility upgrades. As a nation, we have entered a major hospital construction boom. The already strong health care construction sector is projected to grow by 13 percent to a total of $53.8 billion in 2008 and will continue to experience a high growth rate through 2011 (H. Jones, 2007). In the year 2011, this figure is projected to reach $71 billion (FMI, 2007). These forces provide unprecedented opportunities to build better hospitals and renovate existing ones to measurably improve care and working conditions, as well as strengthen their economic well-being.

CONNECTING SAFETY AND QUALITY IMPROVEMENT TO PHYSICAL ENVIRONMENT

Along with the rapid growth in clinical quality improvement research, research on the impacts design can have on safety and quality improvement has also exploded. From 600 articles in 2004 to 1,200 in 2008, the evidence-based design literature provides much to learn (Ulrich and Zimring 2004; Ulrich and Zimring 2008). For example, published research, much of it involving adult patients, tells us that: single patient rooms save lives and reduce harm through fewer infections; wider patient bathroom doors contribute to reducing patient falls; more access to natural light reduces anxiety and depression

---

[1] The Leapfrog Group is a coalition of employers, which have combined their health care purchasing power to reward hospitals that meet certain quality measures. More information is available at www.leapfroggroup.org/home.

[2] In 2003, Centers for Medicare & Medicaid Services and Premier, Inc. hospital alliance partnered to create an innovative quality improvement initiative that provides financial incentives to top performing hospitals based on self-reported quality improvement measures. More information is available at www.premierinc.com/quality-safety/tools-services/p4p/hqi/index.jsp.

[3] More information is available at www.jointcommission.org.

[4] In late 2006, the Institute for Healthcare Improvement launched the national 5 Million Lives Campaign aimed at improving the quality of care and reducing injuries to patients by having hospitals commit to 12 changes: deploy rapid response teams; deliver reliable, evidence-based care for acute myocardial infarction; prevent adverse drug events; prevent central line infections; prevent surgical site infections; prevent ventilator-associated pneumonia; prevent harm from high-alert medications; reduce surgical complications; prevent pressure ulcers; reduce methicillin-resistant staphylococcus aureus infection; deliver reliable, evidence-based care for congestive heart failure; and get boards on board. For more information on these programs, see www.ihi.org.

while shortening length of stay; variable acuity rooms reduce costly, dangerous and unnecessary patient transfers; high efficiency particulate air (HEPA) filtration systems lessen airborne caused infections in immunosupressed patients; and providing positive distractions through music and art can improve the care experience and decrease perception of pain. Some research also shows a clear positive economic effect of evidence-based design.

A significant body of evidence demonstrates that the physical environment is a critical component in any program to improve safety and quality for pediatric patients and provide a safer working environment for the staff who care for them. Children's hospitals' leaders can feel confident that ample evidence supports design decisions for pediatric settings, as well as allows for reasonable extrapolations from adult settings. Lack of evidence is no longer a barrier to incorporating innovation design strategies.

As part of a comprehensive quality improvement program, the physical environment can help to eliminate avoidable conditions such as hospital-acquired infections and must be carefully considered when designing new or renovated facilities (Agency for Healthcare Research and Quality, 2007; Clancy, 2008; Henriksen, Isaacson, Sadler, & Zimring, 2007).

Dr. Carolyn Clancy, director of the Agency for Healthcare Research and Quality (AHRQ) said: "As hospital leaders continue to seek ways to improve quality and reduce errors, it is critical that they look around their own physical environment with the goal of ensuring the hospital contributes to, rather than impedes, the process of healing." AHRQ has developed a video about the importance of good design in contributing to the quality target for boards and hospital leaders and has disseminated the video to over 5,000 U.S. hospitals[5].

When hospital leaders consider reduced operating cost and revenue enhancements, a powerful business case also supports making intelligent evidence-based design decisions. To fully appreciate the revenue implications of evidence-based design, it is important to consider the likely consequences of several major forces changing reimbursement formulas in addition to newly required public reporting of quality/safety outcomes and comparable patient satisfaction scores.

AN APPROACHING FINANCIAL TSUNAMI – PAY FOR PERFORMANCE

In the past few years, a fundamentally new concept has emerged in reimbursement to hospitals and physicians. This is the most significant new reimbursement concept since the enactment of Medicare and Medicaid and the adoption of diagnosis related groups (DRGs). The approach is called value-based purchasing or pay for performance (P4P), and it promises to have a profound impact on the business case for quality improvement, including the physical environment where people work and care is received. Three years ago, CMS and Premier, Inc. launched a major demonstration program involving more than 260 hospitals, which volunteered to submit data on level of compliance with 34 well accepted quality measures that should be performed 100 percent of the time in five high volume clinical focus areas (acute myocardial infarction, coronary artery bypass graft surgery, heart failure, pneumonia, and hip and knee replacement surgery). The program tested the impact of two core concepts — transparency and a potential financial bonus for outstanding performers — on hospital and physician behavior.

---

5 To obtain a copy of the DVD titled "Transforming Hospitals: Designing for Safety and Quality," call AHRQ Publications Clearinghouse at 1-800-358-9295 or e-mail AHRQPubs@ahrq.hhs.gov.

The results were significant with the average hospital compliance score increased by 11.8 percent in the first two years of the program (Premier, Inc., 2006). In addition, the individual scores for the top 50 percentile hospitals are posted on the Premier Web site so consumers can make more informed choices to get the best quality care available[6]. The findings caught the attention of Congress and the nation. While the emphasis so far has been on Medicare patients, it seems safe to assume that Medicaid (the number one volume payer to children's hospitals) and commercial payers will follow in this direction. Indeed, some have already begun.

In 2002, the National Quality Forum (NQF) identified 27 serious reportable events that are largely preventable and should simply never occur in hospitals (National Quality Forum, 2002). This list was updated in 2006 to include 28 events. Building on this work, CMS took the P4P approach to a new level in 2007. CMS selected eight types of occurrences that harm patients and announced that there will be no Medicare reimbursement made for these events if they were caused by the hospital. One of the eight conditions specifically identified is hospital-acquired patient injuries such as those resulting from falls. Several types of hospital-acquired infection are included in the 2007 rule, and several more have been proposed for consideration in 2008 (Revision to Hospital Inpatient Prospective Payment Systems — 2007 FY Occupational Mix Adjustment to Wage Index; Implementation; Final Rule, 2006).

Medicaid programs and commercial payers are already beginning to follow the CMS lead. While the details are far from clear, it seems reasonable to assume that, within three to five years, virtually no payers will reimburse hospitals and physicians for serious harm caused in the facility. Consumers will have easier access to clear, comparable outcome measures and will make choices about where to take their children for care based on this information. Increasingly, consumers will be channeled to payer preferred networks based on quality measures. Poorly performing hospitals could risk losing significant market share. The P4P revolution is gathering momentum.

COMING SOON: HOSPITALS WILL NO LONGER CHARGE FOR THEIR ERRORS

In this new era of transparency and public reporting, hospitals in some states have voluntarily decided not to charge payers and patients for errors caused in the hospital. The connection linking such a policy and an organization's reputation seems obvious. In addition, the connection between hospital errors and the incidence of litigation has been effectively described (Gosfield & Reinertsen, 2005).

Indeed, a no charge policy for hospital-caused errors may soon become standard practice. Hospital associations in Minnesota and Massachusetts have adopted a no charge for errors policy in advance of the CMS rules taking effect, and many other states will likely follow (Beaudoin, 2007). We are entering a new era — one in which patients and payers will no longer tolerate paying for poor performance.

---

6 The Composite Quality Scores for the hospitals performing in the top 50 percentile in each clinical focus area are available at www.premierinc.com.

PATIENT SATISFACTION AND TRANSPARENCY: HCAHPS CHANGES THE RULES

Another significant emerging trend is the mandated reporting of patient experiences in hospitals. With support from CMS and the AHRQ, The Hospital Consumer Assessment of Healthcare Providers and Systems (HCAHPS) survey was developed to: 1) produce comparable data on patients' perspectives of care on topics important to consumers; 2) create incentives through public reporting for hospitals to improve care; and 3) increase public accountability through increased transparency of quality of care. The survey is composed of 27 items, 18 of which encompass critical aspects of the hospital experience, including cleanliness and quietness of the hospital environment and overall rating of the hospital.

Endorsed by NQF and the federal Office of Management and Budget, hospitals subject to the inpatient prospective payment system (IPPS) as of July 2007 must collect and submit HCAHPS data in order to receive their full IPPS annual payment updates (APU) for fiscal year 2008. CMS is connecting data submission with payment and says that those without submitted HCAHPS data may receive an APU reduced by 2 percent (Centers for Medicare & Medicaid Services, 2007). Additionally, HCAHPS data for adult patients has been added to the Hospital Compare Web site in 2008.

While there are no data yet to report on this new trend, it seems reasonable to predict that those hospitals with more comfortable, safe and patient-centered physical environments will be rated higher by patients in the HCAHPS survey. This could significantly influence patient choice of hospitals with a resulting impact on hospital market share and financial bottom line. Indeed, several questions included in HCAHPS relate directly to facility design and healing environments (e.g., quiet environment, cleanliness, timeliness of response to patient calls, communication with providers, pain control). It seems reasonable to assume that Medicaid and commercial payers will again follow the lead of Medicare in linking payment to quality measures, including patient experience with care. Although a similar survey has not yet been developed for children's hospital care, public reporting requirement is a clear trend. Whether or not data are publicly reported, patient and family experiences with care are vital to the hospital's mission and bottom line.

BALANCING ONE-TIME CAPITAL COSTS AND ONGOING OPERATING SAVINGS

With the mounting pressure to improve quality and safety, and the evidence that design of the physical environment can contribute to both, why have all hospitals not rushed to implement evidence-based design innovations such as those described in this book? Some have. For others, the barriers are often thought to be economic — rapidly escalating costs of construction straining or exceeding capital budgets. Incorporating optimal design innovations can cost additional capital dollars initially although many evidence-based design features do not. However, many health care leaders have not realized that over the life of the project, these interventions can also save significant operational costs and far exceed initial incremental capital costs. This lack of awareness is understandable because, until recently, we did not have the evidence to develop solid financial operating impact assessments.

Based on published evidence and actual experience of pioneering health care organizations involved in the Pebble program sponsored by The Center for Health Design, a multidisciplinary team analyzed the data in 2004 and designed the hypothetical Fable Hospital. The non-existing Fable Hospital was conceived as a 300-bed replacement hospital costing $240 million, the average cost of building a hospital at that time. In Fable, the hospital's leaders decided to incorporate all the appropriate, evidence-based design innovations (Berry et al., 2004).

After detailed analysis, estimates including these changes came to a relatively modest one time capital cost of $12 million (or 5 percent of the $240 million base cost). When analyzed, the operating cost savings resulting from reducing infections, eliminating unnecessary patient transfers, minimizing patient falls, lowering drug costs, lessening employee turnover rates, as well as improving market share and philanthropy, are significant. The additional $12 million capital cost would be more than offset by the end of the second year. With effective management and monitoring, the financial operating benefits would continue year after year, making the additional innovations a sound long term investment. In short, there was a compelling business case for building better, safer hospitals. While Fable was largely based on adult patients and research involving adults, the significant majority of components are also relevant to pediatric patients and their hospital environments. The incidence of patient falls and staff lifting injuries are probably the two clearest differences between pediatric and adult environments.

THE COST IMPLICATIONS OF EVIDENCE-BASED DESIGN INNOVATIONS

Since 2004, when the Fable Hospital article made a strong business case for evidence-based environments, considerably more evidence of the impacts of good facility design have amassed, and the cost implications are better understood. Clearly, improved design can lower the life cycle costs of operating hospitals, and many improvements can be made for little or no additional initial cost.

To be sure, the costs of hospital construction have skyrocketed. A combination of increased costs of concrete, steel and other building materials in a competitive global market and the cost of labor and markedly more stringent building code requirements have driven construction and project costs to unprecedented levels. Although this trend is likely to continue for the next five years or more, most experts believe the growth rate will be less dramatic. Despite the substantial construction cost increases, the business case for building better hospitals has become even stronger due to the significant impact of evidence-based design innovations on patient safety and quality and workforce well-being.

As design innovations have been implemented, new information on their cost implications has become available, and guidelines have changed as well. For example, in the United States, single patient rooms have become the standard. They are included in the 2006 American Institute of Architects (AIA) minimum standards, and the advantages are so well documented that they are no longer considered a luxury (Facility Guidelines Institute, AIA Academy of Architecture for Health, and U.S. Department of Health and Human Services, 2006). Because of strong evidence on reduced infections, clear patient preference,

TABLE 4. PENNSYLVANIA HEALTH CARE HOSPITAL-ACQUIRED INFECTION SUMMARY

Case Type	Number of Cases	Mortality Number	Mortality Percent	Average Length of Stay	Average Charge
Hospital-aquired infection	19,154	2,478	12.9%	20.6 days	$185,260
Without hospital-aquired infection	1,550,010	36,238	2.3%	4.5 days	$31,389

improved ability to provide patient centered care and greater efficiency/flexibility in optimal use, single patient rooms are now a basic requirement of most hospitals built today. Failure to follow this standard increasingly places a hospital at a competitive disadvantage in the region and threatens a loss in market share.

Studies show that installing ceiling lifts can significantly reduce the costs of workforce injuries resulting from lifting patients (Chhokar et al., 2005; Joseph & Fritz, 2006). Peace Health in Oregon saw a reduction in the annual cost of patient handling injuries of 83 percent after installing ceiling lifts, resulting in payback on the initial investment in less than two and one-half years (Joseph & Fritz, 2006).

Several new detailed studies document the increased costs, ranging from $8,000 to more than $40,000, incurred for treating patients with hospital-acquired infections (Morrissey, 2004; Murphy & Whiting, 2007; Pennsylvania Health Care Cost Containment Council, 2006). The state of Pennsylvania found that in 2005, 19,154 cases of infection or 12.1 per 1,000 admissions accounted for 394,129 hospital days and $3.5 billion in hospital charges in 168 hospitals. A comparison of cases shows that the charges for patients with hospital-acquired infections were $185,260 compared with $31,389 for patients without an acquired infection. See Table 4. (Pennsylvania Health Care Cost Containment Council, 2006). These studies show that not only does it cost more to treat these patients, but their longer length of stay can also reduce the overall hospital capacity and thus limit the potential to admit new patients. Many indicators suggest that the rate of infection is growing.

Strong evidence suggests that the strategic placement of hand washing dispensers in every patient room and high volume treatment area has become a necessity and should be included in any new or existing hospital as a component to reducing infections (Bischoff, Reynolds, Sessler, Edmond, & Wenzel, 2000; Trick et al., 2007). HEPA filtration systems are effective in reducing airborne-acquired infections and are a worthwhile investment in areas that treat immunocompromised patients (Petska & Young 2006 quoted in Joseph & Fritz, 2006).

Injuries due to patient falls are another cost that will become financially more significant as reimbursement rules change. Ann Hendrich, vice president clinical excellence operations for Ascension Health, estimates the cost per fall to be $19,000, not including the cost of litigation. Research shows that the physical environment is an important component of a program to reduce all falls and can significantly reduce the incidence of patient falls. As such, modifications to the physical environment are among measures recommended by the IHI Transforming Care at the Bedside initiative funded by the Robert Wood Johnson Foundation (Institute for Healthcare Improvement, 2007).

Changes to the physical environment to help reduce falls are not necessarily costly. For instance, larger patient bathrooms with double-door access can be accomplished for as little as $400 per room (Edwards, 2007; Hendrich, Bender, & Nyhuis, 2003). The concept of decentralizing nursing stations to improve sightline visibility to patients and to increase the amount of time for direct patient care has gathered considerable interest. Decentralized nurse stations do not necessarily add overall square footage to facilities and therefore can be cost neutral, as was the case at Dublin Methodist. In the adult environment, reduced patient falls for a 300-bed hospital could result in over $1 million in annual savings. The incidence and cost of falls is presumed to be significantly less in a pediatric population, but it is still important to consider.

The acuity adaptable room is one of the most powerful design innovations and can significantly reduce unnecessary intra-hospital transfers. It offers a threefold benefit of reduced errors and falls, significantly increased patient satisfaction, and reduction in non-productive staff time. While the main study in this area involved adult patients, most of the benefits (reduced errors in handoffs, higher patient and family satisfaction, and reduced unproductive staff) will apply to children's hospitals. As acuity adaptable rooms are adopted, more data on their effect will become available. Dublin Methodist Hospital in Columbus, OH, has assumed the incremental costs of including additional oxygen and vacuum systems in room headwalls is about $5,700 per room, and the possibility of dramatically reducing costly transfers is significant (Edwards, 2007; Ulrich & Zhu, 2007). Significant work in nurse training and culture support is required to realize the benefits made possible by acuity adaptable rooms.

Noise reduction innovations such as acoustical ceiling tiles in patient rooms, corridors and nursing stations are effective economical features. Carpet also effectively reduces noise and can actually cost less than other floor coverings such as vinyl (D. Edwards, personal communication, September 14, 2007). All hospitals should undertake a simple "sound audit" to identify the noisiest areas and adapt simple solutions such as eliminating overhead pagers and moving noisy equipment, which have significant benefits in patient satisfaction (Sharkey, 2007a, 2007b).

Appropriately selected music can also reduce patient anxiety and increase satisfaction with the health care experience. Carefully selected music can reduce stress, enhance a sense of comfort and relaxation, offer distraction from pain, and enhance clinical performance (Kemper & Danhauer, 2005). Music can also reduce the need for anesthesia in certain circumstances. In the pediatric unit of Tallahassee Memorial Hospital, a specially trained musician interacted with pediatric patients scheduled for echocardiograms or computed tomography scans. The calming effect eliminated the need for anesthesia in over 90 percent of the procedures (DeLoach Walworth, 2005).

Many well designed innovations involving music and the arts have shown measurable positive influence in reducing anxiety, stress and sleep deprivation and improving patient perceptions of their experience. Most of these interventions are extremely low cost and can be implemented by any hospital. In addition, funding for these projects can frequently be provided by philanthropy from the arts community, so they do not compete with other philanthropic needs of the hospital.

An improved, quieter work environment can also reduce stress and contribute to improved nurse satisfaction scores (PricewaterhouseCoopers LLP, University of Sheffield, & Queen Margaret University College - Edinburgh, 2004). The need to reduce employee turnover and improve retention has never been greater. A recent detailed and thorough calculation of nursing turnover estimates the cost of loss per registered nurse between $62,100 and $67,100 (C. B. Jones, 2005). This study calculated the actual costs from four hospitals, including the costs of advertising, hiring temporary staff, training, and reduced productivity.

Evidence-based design interventions measurably reduce operating costs and, by increasing patient/family satisfaction, can increase market share. They provide concrete examples for children's hospitals to consider when making building decisions.

GOING GREEN: ANOTHER DIMENSION OF THE BUSINESS CASE

In addition to evidence-based design features that address patient and staff safety, a number of emerging sustainable or "green" building features and strategies can improve the health care environment with little or no capital cost and should be considered for inclusion in new projects. Sustainable design is increasingly recognized as a key component of the hospital safety agenda. In addition, incorporating proven green building features establishes a hospital as a good community partner in improving the overall environment.

At the end of 2007, a coalition of large hospital systems and nonprofit organizations created the Global Health and Safety Initiative specifically to address the triple safety agendas of patients, workers and the environment. While a comprehensive review of sustainability features appropriate for health care design is beyond the scope of this chapter, hospital leaders should be aware of the relationship to the business case. A detailed examination of sustainability in health care facilities was recently published by Robin Guenther and Gail Vittori (2008).

Similar to the evidence-based design features discussed above, sustainable design does not necessarily have a cost premium. The most widely cited study of green building, conducted by Gregory Kats, found that green office and school buildings have, on average, a 2 percent capital cost premium, which was more than recovered though operational savings – primarily energy and water savings (2003). Moreover, green buildings may well deliver health and productivity benefits that standard buildings, known as "brown buildings," do not. Kats' research in the office and school sectors correlate improved productivity and reduced absenteeism with green buildings, and both can be translated to cost savings.

While no definitive study of the cost of green hospital buildings has been published at this writing, the cost-consulting firm Davis Langdon recently published the "Cost of Green Revisited" comparing the capital cost of green and brown ambulatory care facilities in California (Matthiessen & Morris, 2007). The study found that green ambulatory care facilities are not distinguishable in capital cost from their brown counterparts. There are low cost and high cost green buildings, just as there are low cost and high cost brown buildings. Ultimately, capital cost differences related to building type in a geographic area are attributable to program issues, team experience, site factors and a range of other local factors.

In addition to the obvious financial benefits associated with energy and water reduction, green buildings incorporate innovative materials and products proving to reduce the operational cost of buildings. Green materials often have performance benefits above and beyond their environmental attributes, as manufacturers have been reluctant to introduce green products at premium pricing unless they have additional improvements. Rubber flooring exemplifies a product that can have benefits to the bottom line, the environment and make for a safer and better performing hospital. Kaiser Permanente and Herman Miller have found that the initial cost premium compared to the cost of standard vinyl flooring is offset by a combination of reduced maintenance costs and improved safety. The environmental benefit is that it replaces polyvinyl chloride, which links to detrimental health effects and must be maintained by labor intensive waxing and stripping protocols and negatively affects indoor air quality. Additional benefits arise from improved traction (reduced slip and fall) and noise dampening, which creates a more tranquil environment (Fudge, 2006). Plus, it is softer under foot, reducing strain on caregivers who walk miles per shift.

Many green strategies improving indoor air quality have no cost premium at all and just require thoughtful selection and procedures. Material finishes with low volatile organic compound (VOC) emissions are readily available at little if any additional cost. As green building becomes more pervasive, the range of product offerings increase, and cost premiums associated with innovation give way to the competition of the marketplace.

Finally, a number of strategies can intersect to reduce initial construction cost and may yield unanticipated benefits. At Modesto Hospital, for example, Kaiser Permanente found installation of porous paving less expensive because porous paving allows storm water to move directly through the surface of the pavement to join groundwater beneath (Guenther & Vittori, 2008). The savings accrued from eliminating the underground storm water conveyance system more than covered the premium associated with the porous pavement. An additional unanticipated benefit is no wet feet on rainy days, reducing slips and falls in the lobby.

Including emerging new evidence relating to green, sustainable buildings should become an important ingredient in any business case analysis.

A CHALLENGE: CONVERTING "LIGHT GREEN" TO "DARK GREEN" DOLLARS

To realize all the financial benefits of the green analysis, it is essential to make cultural and operational changes in tandem with changes to the physical environment. For example, reducing intrahospital transfers through variable acuity rooms will not occur through physical environment changes alone; significant investment in culture and training must be made and implemented. Decreasing the number of transfers will have significant patient satisfaction benefits and reduce errors, but it won't produce efficiency savings at the bottom line unless staffing levels are adjusted downwards, thus reducing labor costs.

To fully document the business case, costs avoided by reducing infections or patient falls must be estimated, captured and reflected in the organization's financial statements. Similarly, costs avoided by reducing nursing turnover must be captured by estimating the savings in recruitment and training.

Moving theoretical savings (light green dollars) to actual savings and reflecting it in the hospital financial statements (dark green dollars) is a key success factor to accomplish objectives of the business case. An interdisciplinary team at IHI first described this business case objective, which is true of quality improvement innovations as well as environmental changes (Nolan & Bisognano, 2006). Documenting actual cost savings is invaluable in convincing boards of trustees that evidence-based design investments are cost effective.

MAKING IT HAPPEN: ASK QUESTION NUMBER 6

Traditionally, hospital leaders have asked five questions when considering a major building project:
1. Urgency – Is the expansion or replacement actually needed now to fulfill the hospital's mission? What is the cost strategically of not proceeding?
2. Appropriateness – Is the proposed plan the most reasonable and prudent in light of other alternatives?
3. Cost – Is the cost per square foot appropriate in light of other projects being built in the region?
4. Financial impact – Has the financial impact of additional volume, depreciation expense and revenue assumptions been reasonably analyzed and projected?
5. Sources of funds – Is the anticipated combination of additional operating income, reserves, borrowing and philanthropy reasonable and enough to support the project?

However, hospitals leaders should also address a sixth question:
6. Evidence-based design – Will the proposed project incorporate all relevant evidence-based design innovations in order to optimize patient safety, quality and satisfaction as well as workforce safety, productivity and energy efficiency?

As hospital leaders undertake building projects, it is imperative that the ongoing operating savings be an integral part of the analysis (Sadler, 2006a). Hospital boards must hold management accountable to new levels of environmental excellence and efficiency. Building a new hospital or undertaking a major renovation is likely the biggest financial decision that a board will ever make. It also provides a unique opportunity to transform the culture and processes of the overall organization (Hamilton and Orr, 2008). Indeed, major changes in culture and organizational processes are essential if the benefits of an improved physical environment are to be realized.

FROM IDEAS TO ACTION: TEN STEPS TO CREATE YOUR BUSINESS CASE

Hospitals typically undertake a comprehensive financial analysis before committing to a major project, including asking the five basic questions. To address question number six effectively, financial assumptions about the impact of evidence-based design interventions should be developed. Management and the board must commit to measure and record potential outcomes for these financial impacts. The chief financial officer must play a leadership role in this effort.

Effectively incorporating evidence-based design will require leadership to undertake at least the following 10 steps:
1. *Create a multidisciplinary leadership team.* Management, medical staff and board leaders must work as a team to develop a common vision with specific goals, including volume and quality improvements, to achieve in the new project.
2. *Choose the right architects.* Select architects with a proven understanding of and experience in evidence-based design. Look for actual examples of how an architect has incorporated evidence-based design innovations in completed or planned projects. Look for certification like Evidence-Based Design Assessment and Certification

developed by The Center for Health Design, which educates and assesses individuals on their understanding of how to base design decisions on available, credible evidence.

3. *Identify evidence-based design interventions.* Architects, management, medical staff and board leadership must collaborate to determine which cost effective evidence-based design interventions will support their vision for the new project.

4. *Evaluate current practices and develop a baseline for each.* For example, determine institutionally and at the patient unit level the current rates of transfers, employee turnover and patient falls. Identify the baseline operating costs associated with these outcomes.

5. *Set measurable post-occupancy improvement targets.* For example, establish targets for a reduction in hospital-acquired infections from X to Y; an increase in patient satisfaction rates from A to B; decrease in workforce lift injuries from C to D; and reduction in patient transfers from E to F. These measurable improvement targets must be agreed to by all key stakeholders and communicated widely. To be successful, it is essential to build an organizational culture of support for these changes, including enthusiastic staff leaders who are strong advocates (Hamilton, Orr, & Raboin, 2008, in press).

6. *Incorporate design innovations within capital and operating budgets.* Management and medical leadership must incorporate the financial impact of these improvements into the hospital's annual capital and operating budgets, which are reviewed and approved by the board of trustees.

7. *Communicate improvement targets.* Performance improvement targets including the methods used to collect data should be included in all appropriate internal and external communications. Public awareness and recognition can differentiate the organization in the marketplace and increase market share.

8. *Track and report progress.* When the new facility or renovation opens, the metrics of impact (including financial impact) at the overall institutional level and the unit level should be regularly reported to all key stakeholders, including the board.

9. *Continually incorporate new evidence-based design.* Regularly review internal experience and new developments in evidence-based design. Where appropriate, incorporate new evidence-based design interventions into the facility maintenance activities, process and culture. While tracking of impact should continue for at least two years post-occupancy, emerging environmental design and process improvements should be systematically incorporated.

10. *Publish your results.* The organization should commit to sharing lessons learned and publishing the results, including financial impacts. Continuing the conversation with the design community will contribute to needed knowledge about the financial impact of evidence-based design.

(This analysis is drawn from the article by Sadler, DuBose and Zimring, "The Business Case for Building Better Hospitals Through Evidence-based Design," Health Environments Research and Design Journal, June 2008.)

TABLE 5: PROBLEM SCOPE AND IMPROVEMENT OPPORTUNITY

Outcome	Number of cases	Rate per 1,000 admissions	Average hospital cost per admission
Hospital-acquired infections		(Number of hospital-acquired infections cases / total admissions) x 1,000	
No hospital-acquired infections		(Number of no hospital-acquired infections cases / total admissions) x 1,000	
Total admissions			
Incremental cost for all hospital-acquired infections cases			Average cost hospital-acquired infections minus average cost no hospital-acquired infections
Incremental cost for hospital-acquired infections cases			Average cost unreimbursed hospital-acquired infections minus average cost no hospital-acquired infections

A FRAMEWORK FOR EVALUATING EVIDENCE-BASED DESIGN FEATURES

The following return on investment framework can help establish the business case to evaluate specific evidence-based design innovations (E. Malone, unpublished Return on Investment Framework for Evaluating Evidence-based Design Features, 2008). Each organization will need to incorporate the latest evidence and its best judgment about the impact of design innovations on cost and revenue.

For example, a business plan for reducing hospital-acquired infections, would require defining the scope of the problem, targeting improvement goals, planning clinical and administrative interventions and understanding how evidence-based design would contribute to the solution. Both initial and life cycle incremental costs and/or savings are provided for all interventions to allow comparison between cost of intervention and the financial benefit associated with avoiding certain costs. The framework should work equally well for other evidence-based design innovations.

Goal: Reduce hospital-acquired infections

This return on investment framework contains four steps. Tables are provided to assist with managing data collection, calculation and analysis.

Step 1: Identify scope of the problem and improvement opportunity. Describe the current extent of the problem by gathering data and calculating impact using Table 5.
- Identify total admissions for the previous year. Consider capturing these data for several years to develop an average baseline or trend
- From total admissions, determine how many patients contracted hospital-acquired infections[7]
- Identify average hospital cost per admission for patients with and without hospital-acquired infections
- Identify your improvement goal, for example, reduce hospital-acquired infections to X number per year

---

[7] A guideline to identifying patients with hospital-acquired infections can be found in the Pennsylvania Cost Containment Council Report technical section, found at www.phc4.org/reports/hai/

TABLE 6: IMPROVEMENT COSTS SUMMARY

Intervention	Initial cost	Annual cost
Provide 100% single patient rooms	Single patient rooms are now the standard for new hospital construction, therefore no additional cost is assumed	No additional cost assumed
Separate sink for staff in patient room	Separate staff sinks are now considered standard for new hospital construction, therefore no additional cost assumed	No additional cost assumed
Alcohol-based gel devices	Cost of device x additional number of devices per room x number of rooms	Replacement, maintenance and gel refill costs
Increased HEPA filtration	Incremental cost of HEPA capable air handlers x number of air handlers	Increased energy and incremental filter replacement cost
Clinical and administrative interventions (e.g., education)	Training program and educational materials	New employee training and evaluation of compliance
Total cost of improvements		

TABLE 7: REVENUE IMPROVEMENT

Avoided hospital-acquired infections cases	Incremental cost per hospital-acquired infection	Annual cost avoidance
Baseline number of hospital-acquired infections minus targeted number of hospital-acquired infections		Avoided hospital-acquired infections cases x incremental cost per hospital-acquired infections case

TABLE 8: RETURN ON INVESTMENT

Variables	Initial year	Year two	Year five
Cumulative cost avoidance	Annual cost avoidance	Annual cost avoidance x 2	Annual cost avoidance x 5
Cumulative cost of improvements	Initial cost	Initial cost + annual cost	Initial cost + (annual cost x 4)
Savings	Cost avoidance minus cost of improvements	Cost avoidance minus cost of improvements	Cost avoidance minus cost of improvements

Step 2: Estimate improvement costs. Identify the specific evidence-based design strategies as well as clinical and administrative strategies that you will use to reach your goal, and identify associated initial and life-cycle costs (Table 6).

Examples of evidence-based design interventions include:
- Create 100 percent single patient rooms
- Ensure that there are separate hand washing sinks for staff in patient rooms and that the sinks are unavoidably visible and available
- Provide alcohol-based hand gel disinfection devices in multiple locations in patient rooms, such as on either side of the patient's bed, in the family zone of the patient's room and in the patient's bathroom
- Install HEPA filters in ventilation system

Examples of clinical and administrative strategies are:
- Educate staff, patients and visitors about organizational patient safety priority of reducing hospital-acquired infections
- Actively identify patients who carry multi-drug resistant organisms
- Use contact and equipment precautions for all multi-drug resistant patients
- Ensure that the environmental cleaning plan includes all surfaces in close proximity to patients and frequently touched surfaces on a more frequent cleaning schedule for known multi-drug resistant patients

Step 3: Revenue improvement through cost avoidance. Identify the potential savings associated with reducing hospital-acquired infections. Using figures calculated in Step 1, determine the annual cost avoided if the hospital-acquired infections goal is achieved (Table 7). Consider calculating an average number of hospital-acquired infections cases to develop a baseline number or consider using the figure from the previous year. If the hospital census has changed dramatically, consider using the rate of hospital-acquired infections instead of the absolute number.

Step 4: Calculate the return on investment. Compare the total annual cost avoidance identified in Step 3 with the total initial cost of the planned interventions in Step 2 to identify the financial savings over interim points along the hospital life cycle (Table 8). For years two and five, assume the same annual costs and cost avoidance for each year or adjust costs adjusted for inflation.

THE BUSINESS CASE FOR BUILDING BETTER PEDIATRIC FACILITIES APPENDIX

FOUR CASE STUDIES

The following four case studies demonstrate how different organizations have successfully incorporated evidence-based design into capital projects. The first two describe specific design innovations in completed projects showing significant measurable economic benefit. The third and fourth describe clear commitments to incorporate evidence-based design in all new military health facilities and into a new children's hospital.

Peace Health Medical Center in Eugene, OR

Like most hospitals, Peace Health Medical Center (PHMC) confronted a significant number of back injuries to nurses involved in lifting and moving patients. The hospital explored several mechanical devices being tested in concert with a "no manual lift" policy.

Based on the evidence available about the benefits of using ceiling lifts, the hospital installed ceiling lifts in 26 of 33 intensive care units (ICU) rooms in late 2002 and in all 24 neurology rooms in late 2003. Incident reports obtained from both units spanned a period of 60 months (January 2001 to December 2006). The ICU had 10 injuries related to patient handling in the two years before installation of ceiling lifts. Annual cost of patient handling injuries was $142,500. After lifts were installed in more than 75 percent of the rooms, there were no injuries during the study period caused by moving patients using the lifts (Joseph & Fritz, 2006).

In neurology, there were 15 injuries related to patient handling in the three years before installation of ceiling lifts. The annual cost of patient handling injuries in this unit was $222,645. In the two years since installation on the unit, there have been six injuries, some with extenuating circumstances (e.g., failure to use the lift or a combative patient). The annual cost in neurology after lift installation was $54,660.

Peace Health is building a new replacement hospital. Based on the dramatic findings of the study, it will make 309 rooms lift ready and will install 234 transverse rails and lifts. It expects to get a return on investment in two and one-half years in the new facility. The authors conclude: "With Peace Health's new ergonomics program in place and 100 percent compliance in using ceiling lifts, the savings could be phenomenal" (Joseph & Fritz, 2006).

Methodist Hospital, Clarian Health Partners, Inc., Indianapolis, IN

Clarian recognized that delayed transfers of patients between nursing units and lack of available beds are significant problems that increase costs and decrease quality of care and satisfaction among patients and staff. Patients are transferred as often as three to six times during their stays to match care needs with level of acuity. In a pioneering project, a team led by Ann Hendrich, vice president clinical excellence operations for Ascension Health, replaced a multilevel ICU with single variable acuity adaptable rooms. In designing the new 56-bed ICU (28 rooms on two floors), each single room was equipped with an acuity adaptable headwall, equipped with the gases and equipment needed to adjust with patient acuity.

Twelve outcome-based questions were formulated. Two years of baseline data were collected before the unit moved and were compared with three years of data collected after the move.

The team found significant improvement postmove in key areas: patient transfers decreased by 90 percent, medication errors by 70 percent, and number of falls decreased drastically. Run charts are included in the published article (Hendrich, Fay, & Sorrells, 2004). The costs savings are significant and make a strong business case for this approach.

APPENDIX | THE BUSINESS CASE FOR BUILDING BETTER PEDIATRIC FACILITIES | 113

The Military Health System

The Military Health System (MHS) provides care to 9.2 million beneficiaries with approximately 130,000 staff in 70 military hospitals, 411 primary care clinics and 417 dental clinics around the world. Consequent to several recently enacted laws, including the 2006 Base Realignment and Closure Act, the military plans to increase the number of serving soldiers and Marines and to move some military units back to the United States. The MHS finds itself with a $6 billion portfolio of health care facility projects planned over the next five years. These projects include closing historic Walter Reed Army Medical Center and merging its mission with the National Naval Medical Center to create the Walter Reed National Military Medical Center in Bethesda, MD, and a new robust community hospital at Fort Belvoir in Northern Virginia to serve the almost half a million beneficiaries in the nation's capital region. As a result of these and other health facility projects, MHS finds itself with a once-in-a-lifetime opportunity to transform its worldwide health care infrastructure and contribute to the body of evidence-based design science. Embracing evidence-based design will set the stage to support the outcomes our soldiers and their families deserve. So how is MHS organized to succeed?

TABLE D

Military Health System Evidence-based Design Principles and Goals

Create a Patient and Family Centered Environment Reflecting the MHS Culture of Caring

- Increase social support
- Reduce special disorientation
- Improve patient privacy and confidentiality
- Provide adequate and appropriate light exposure
- Support optimal patient nutrition
- Improve patient sleep and rest
- Decrease exposure to harmful chemicals

Improve the Quality and Safety of Health Care

- Reduce hospital-acquired infections via airborne, contact and water routes of transmission
- Reduce medication errors
- Prevent patient falls
- Reduce noise stress and improve speech intelligibility

Enhance Care of the Whole Person by Providing Contact with Nature and Positive Distractions

- Decrease patient and family stress

Create a Positive Work Environment

- Decrease back pain and work-related injuries
- Reduce staff fatigue
- Increase team effectiveness
- Eliminate noisy and chaotic environments

Design for Maximum Standardization, Future Flexibility and Growth

- Reduce room transfers
- Facilitate care coordination and patient service

All transformational endeavors require leaders who can envision the future, articulate the goals and mobilize the organization to reshape its culture and processes. The MHS launched the evidence-based design campaign in January 2007 with clear direction from the assistant secretary for defense for health affairs who directed the Army Corps of Engineers and the Navy Facilities Engineering Command: "[I]nstruct the respective design teams to apply patient centered and evidence-based design principles across all medical construction projects. A growing body of research has demonstrated that the built environment can positively influence health outcomes, patient safety and long-term operating efficiencies to include reduction in staff injuries, reduction in nosocomial infection rates, patient falls and reductions in length of hospital stay. Incorporating the results of this research along with changes in concepts of operations into the design of some of its most significant facilities will allow the MHS and the patients entrusted to our care to reap substantial health and system wide benefits for many years to come (Malone, Mann-Dooks & Strauss (2007)."

The MHS evidence-based design team, comprised doctors, nurses, administrators, architects and engineers engaged in a deliberate planning process that resulted in the creation of an evidence-based design road map, which includes principles, goals and desired outcomes linked to the larger MHS strategic plan and specifies the recommended evidence-based design features and responses (Malone, Mann-Dooks, & Strauss, 2007). A summary of the MHS evidence-based design principles and subsequent goals are in Table D (previous page).

Evidence-based design activities currently engaged in by MHS include:
- Engaging senior leaders to provide transformation leadership
- Partnering with clinical and administrative peers to lead necessary clinical and business process re-engineering
- Including patients and family members in all aspects of facility planning
- Refining evidence-based design cost estimating to include return-on-investment analysis that links features in the built environment with improvements in patient and staff safety and quality of care, staff satisfaction and improvements to the bottom line
- Reviewing and restructuring acquisition processes to streamline the delivery of projects with evidence-based design features
- Reviewing outcome metrics definitions and methodology to ensure comparability on a national level
- Engaging the research teams to focus on replicating previous studies in the inpatient environment as well as initiating new evidence-based design research across the health care continuum, with particular focus on ambulatory care and dental environments
- Harvesting emerging evidence-based design application tools and lessons learned
- Disseminating evidence-based design information
- Refining the post-occupancy evaluation process
- Publishing and sharing evidence-based design experiences and lessons learned

Engaged and focused leadership fuels and focuses cross-pollination and drives disciplined execution at every step in the process by setting the vision and then coaching, managing and rewarding the team engaged in the work of cultural and process re-engineering. Well conceived strategies will fail without transformational leaders and disciplined execution.

The stakes could not be higher, as the current MHS, Assistant Secretary for Defense for Health Affairs S. Ward Casscells, M.D., reminds us, "… the best isn't good enough for our warriors. Nothing short of excellence is good enough for these patients and their families. We have an unprecedented opportunity to modernize many of our key facilities over the next five years. We can and must ensure that our hospital designs promote integrity during the clinical encounter … empower our patients and families … relieve suffering … and promote long-term health and wellness (Casscell, 2008)."

Systems improvement represents a complex poetry that demands leader-driven engagement to solve the challenging problems facing health care today (Berwick, 2007).

The Children's Hospital, Aurora, CO
Due to a military base closure, The Children's Hospital, Aurora, CO, was given the chance to build a total replacement pediatric hospital on a green field site. This presented a once-in-a-lifetime opportunity to evaluate the outcomes of a facility designed and built with the best available evidence.

The purpose of the research study is to evaluate and compare the impact of the original and newly built hospital environments on patients, families and staff.

Specific aims:
- Measure family and staff satisfaction with light, noise, temperature, aesthetics and amenities
- Evaluate staff and family perceptions of safety, security and privacy
- Compare nosocomial infection rates between the old and new facilities
- Track work flow and staff efficiency
- Examine correlations between private/semi-private rooms and clinical outcomes
- Assess family use of overnight facilities

Using pre and post-surveys, all nursing, social work, therapy, housekeeping staff and families on selected inpatient units are invited to participate. A brief demographic form, the Work Environment Scale (Moos, 1994), a Family and Staff Satisfaction Survey, and selected questions from the Press, Ganey Inpatient Pediatric Survey will be analyzed pre- and post-relocation. Data on nosocomial infection rates, staffing (ratios and turnover), work flow, skill mix and variance reports also will be collected. The hospital collected data in the original facility both six months prior to its move and six months post-move. It will collect again at 12 months post-move.

Children's Hospital expects families and staff to report greater satisfaction with hospital aesthetics and amenities, environmental safety and security, and parking and way-finding at the new facility compared to the original hospital. Families will report more privacy, less noise and better temperature regulation in the new private rooms versus the semi-private rooms of the original facility. Children in private rooms will experience fewer nosocomial infections, medication errors and falls, shorter lengths of stay, and greater satisfaction with pain management than children in semi-private rooms. Decentralized caregiver stations will increase staff nurse efficiency and bedside presence and improve work flow compared to centralized caregiver stations.

Several initial findings have surfaced, but none more dramatic than the change in staff turnover. The pre-move turnover data from October 2007 reflected a nurse turnover annualized percentage of 9.55 percent. The March 2008 nursing turnover rate, six months post-move, is 4.38 percent. These rates are significant when compared to the national turnover rate estimated at 15 percent. This dramatic result shows that Children's Hospital was able to achieve its stated goal of attracting and retaining staff. Future measurement and data collection will help to document the impact of the facility on the nurse retention improvement and other outcomes of the new Children's Hospital.

REFERENCES CITED

Ackerman, B., Sherwonit, E., & Fisk, W. (1989). Reduced incidental light exposure: Effect on the development of retinopathy of prematurity in low birth weight infants. *Pediatrics, 83*(6), 958-962.

Agency for Healthcare Research and Quality. (2007). Transforming hospitals: Designing for safety and quality. DVD.

Al-Samsam, R., & Cullen, O. (2005). Sleep and adverse environmental factors in sedated, mechanically ventilated pediatric intensive care patients. *Pediatric Critical Care Medicine, 6*(5), 562-567.

Altimier, L. B. (2004). Healing environments: for patients and providers. *Newborn & Infant Nursing Reviews, 4*(2), 89-92.

Alton, M., Frush, K., Brandon, D., & Mericle, J. (2006). Development and implementation of a pediatric patient safety program. *Advances in Neonatal Care.*

Archibald, L. K., Manning, M. L., Bell, L. M., Banerjee, S., & Jarvis, W. R. (1997). Patient density, nurse-to-patient ratio and nosocomial infection risk in a pediatric cardiac intensive care unit. *The Pediatric Infectious Disease Journal, 16*(11), 1045-1048.

Arnon, S., Shapsa, A., Forman, L., Regev, R., Bauer, S., Litmanovitz, I., et al. (2006). Live music is beneficial to preterm infants in the neonatal intensive care unit environment. *Birth, 33*(2), 131-136.

Avila-Aguero, M., German, G., Paris, M., Herrera, J., & Group, S. T. S. (2004). Toys in a pediatric hospital: Are they a bacterial source? *American Journal of Infection Control 32*(5), 287-290.

Ayako, N., Mitsuru, S., Yoshitaka, T., & Tsutomu, Y. (2002). Architectural planning of children's hospital wards from a point of view of play environment as assessed by children. *Journal of Architecture, Planning, and Environmental Engineering,* 113-120.

Baehr, E., Fogg, L. F., & Eastman, C. I. (1999). Intermittent bright light and exercise to entrain human circadian rhythms to night work. *American Journal of Physiology, 277,* 1598-1604.

Bailey, E., & Timmons, S. (2005). Noise levels in PICU: An evaluative study. *Paediatric Nursing, 17*(10), 22-26.

Batista-Miranda, J., Darbey, M., Kelly, M., & Baurer, S. (1995). Environment, patient, information, and organization in a pediatrics urodynamics unit. *Arch Esp Urol, 48*(1), 15-22.

Battles, H., & Wiener, L. (2002). Starbright World: Effects of an electronic network on the social environment of children with life-threatening illnesses. *Children's Health Care, 31*(1), 47-68.

Bayo, M. V., Garcia, A. M., & Garcia, A. (1995). Noise levels in an urban hospital and workers' subjective responses. *Archives of Environmental Health, 50*(3), 247-251.

Beauchemin, K. M., & Hays, P. (1996). Sunny hospital rooms expedite recovery from severe and refractory depressions. *Journal of Affective Disorders, 40*(1-2), 49-51.

Beaudoin, J. (2007, November 20). Massachusetts hospitals make "no charge" pledge for adverse events. *Healthcare Finance News.*

Becker, F. (2007). The ecology of knowledge networks. *California Management Review, 49*(2), 1-20.

Bellieni, C. V., Buonocore, G., Pinto, I., Stacchini, N., Cordelli, D. M., & Bagnoli, F. (2003). Use of sound-absorbing panel to reduce noisy incubator reverberating effects. *Biol Neonate, 84*(4), 293-296.

Ben-Abraham, R., Keller, N., Szold, O., Vardi, A., Weinberg, M., Barzilay, Z., et al. (2002). Do isolation rooms reduce the rate of nosocomial infections in the pediatric intensive care unit? *Journal of Critical Care, 17*(3), 176-180.

Benedetti, F., Colombo, C., Barbini, B., Campori, E., & Smeraldi, E. (2001). Morning sunlight reduces length of hospitalization in bipolar depression. *Journal of Affective Disorders, 62*(3), 221-223.

Berens, R. (1999). Noise in the pediatric intensive care unit. *Journal of Intensive Care Medicine, 14*(3), 118-129.

Berens, R. J. & Weigle, C. G. (1996). Cost analysis of ceiling tile replacement for noise abatement. *Journal of Perinatology, 16*(3 Pt 1), 199-201.

Berry, L., Parker, D., Coile, R., Hamilton, D. K., O'Neill, D., & Sadler, B. (2004). The business case for better buildings. *Frontiers in Health Services Management, 21*(1), 3-21.

Bers, M., Gonzalez-Heydrich, J., & DeMaso, D. (2003). Use of a computer-based application in a pediatric hemodialysis unit: A pilot study. *Journal of the American Academy of Child and Adolescent Psychiatry, 42*(4), 493-496.

Bers, M., Gonzalez-Heydrich, J., Raches, D., & DeMaso, D. (2001). Zora: A pilot virtual community in the pediatric dialysis unit. *Medinfo, 10*(Part 1), 800-804.

Berwick, D. M. (2007). Eating Soup with a Fork. Plenary presentation at the 19th Annual Forum on Quality Improvement in Healthcare.

Bischoff, W. E., Reynolds, T. M., Sessler, C. N., Edmond, M. B., & Wenzel, R. P. (2000). Handwashing compliance by health care workers: The impact of introducing an accessible, alcohol-based hand antiseptic. *Archives of Internal Medicine, 160*(7), 1017-1021.

Blackburn, S. & Patteson, D. (1991). Effects of cycled light on activity state and cardiorespiratory function in preterm infants. *Journal of Perinatal & Neonatal Nursing, 4(*4), 47-54.

Blomkvist, V., Eriksen, C. A., Theorell, T., Ulrich, R. S., & Rasmanis, G. (2005). Acoustics and psychosocial environment in coronary intensive care. *Occupational and Environmental Medicine, 62,* 1-8.

Blumberg, R. & Devlin, A. S. (2006). Design issues in hospitals: The adolescent client. *Environment and Behavior, 38*(3), 293-317.

Boivin, D. & James, F. (2002). Circadian adaptation to night-shift work by judicious light and darkness exposure. *Journal of Biological Rhythms, 17*(6), 556-567.

Bouchard, F., Landry, M., Belles-Isles, M., & Gagnon, J. (2004). A magical dream: A pilot project in animal-assisted therapy in pediatric oncology. *Cancer Oncology Nursing, 14*(1), 14-17.

Bowie, B. H., Hall, R. B., Faulkner, J., & Anderson, B. (2003). Single-room infant care: Future trends in special care nursery planning and design. *Neonatal Network, 22*(4), 27-34.

Boyce, P., Hunter, C., & Howlett, O. (2003). *The benefits of daylight through windows.* Troy, New York: Rensselaer Polytechnic Institute.

Boyd, J., & Hunsberger, M. (1998). Chronically ill children coping with repeated hospitalizations: Their perceptions and suggested interventions. *Journal of Pediatric Nursing, 13*(6), 330-342.

Brady, M. T. (2005). Health care-associated infections in the neonatal intensive care unit. *American Journal of Infection Control, 33*(5), 268-275.

Brandon, D. H., Holditch-Davis, D., & Belyea, M. (2002). Preterm infants born at less than 31 weeks gestation have improved growth in cycled light compared with continuous near darkness. *The Journal of Pediatrics, 140*(2), 192-199.

Bremmer, P., Byers, J., & Kiehl, E. (2003). Noise and the premature infant: Physiological effects and practice implications. *Journal of Obstetric, Gynecologic, and Neonatal Nursing, 32*(4), 447-454.

Brice, J., & Barclay, L. (2007). Music eases anxiety of children in cast room. *Journal of Pediatric Orthopedics, 27,* 831-833.

Brodie, S., Biley, F., & Shewring, M. (2002). An exploration of the potential risks associated with using pet therapy in healthcare settings. *Journal of Clinical Nursing, 11*(4), 444-456.

Brokstein, R., Cohen, S., & Walco, G. (2002). Starbright World and psychological adjustment in children with cancer: A clinical series. *Children's Health Care, 31*(1), 29-45.

Brophy, M. O. R., Achimore, L., & Moore-Dawson, J. (2001). Reducing incidence of low-back injuries reduces cost. *American Industrial Hygiene Association Journal, 62*(4), 508.

Buchanan, T. L., Barker, K. N., Gibson, J. T., Jiang, B. C., & Pearson, R. E. (1991). Illumination and errors in dispensing. *American Journal of Hospital Pharmacy, 48*(10), 2137-2145.

Buick, M. (2007). *Fall prevention is a team effort: Strategies to reduce pediatric falls.* Paper presented at the NACHRI & N.A.C.H. 2007 Creating Connections Conference.

Burgio, L., Engel, B., Hawkins, A., McCorick, K., & Scheve, A. (1990). A descriptive analysis of nursing staff behaviors in a teaching nursing home: Differences among NAs, LPNs and RNs. *The Gerontologist, 30,* 107-112.

Bush, J. P., Huchital, J. R., & Simonian, S. J. (2002). An introduction to program and research initiatives of the Starbright Foundation. *Children's Health Care, 31*(1), 1-10.

Buttery, J., Alabaster, S., Heine, R., Scott, S., Cruchfield, R., Bigham, A., et al. (1999). Multiresistant psuedomonas aeruginosa outbreak in a pediatric oncology ward related to bath toys. *Pediatric Infectious Disease Journal, 17*(6), 509-513.

Byers, J. F., Waugh, W. R., & Lowman, L. B. (2006). Sound level exposure of high-risk infants in different environmental conditions. *Neonatal Network: NN, 25*(1), 25-32.

Caprilli, S. & Messeri, A. (2006). Animal-assisted activity at A. Meyer Children's Hospital: A pilot study. *Evidence Based Complementary and Alternative Medicine, 3*(3), 179-183.

Carney, T., Murphy, S., McClure, J., Bishop, E., Kerr, C., Parker, J., et al. (2003). Children's views of hospitalization: An exploratory study of data collection. *Journal of Child Health Care, 7*(1), 27-40.

Carpman, J. & Grant, M. (1993). *Design that cares: Planning health facilities for patients and visitors* (2nd Edition ed.). Chicago: American Hospital Pub.

Carvalho, A. M. & Begnis, J. G. (2006). Play in pediatric care units: Applications and perspectives. *Psicologia em Estudo, 11*(1), 109-117.

Casscell, W. S. (2008). *A clean sheet of paper.* Paper presented at the 2008 Annual Military Health System Conference.

Centers for Medicare & Medicaid Services. (2007). Hospital care quality information from the consumer perspective. Retrieved January 10, 2008, from http://www.hcahpsonline.org/default.aspx.

Chaberny, I., Schnitzler, P., Geiss, H., & Wendt, C. (2003). An outbreak of epidemic keratoconjunctivitis in a pediatric unit due to Adenovirus type 8. *Infection Control and Hospital Epidemiology, 24,* 514-519.

Chang, Y.-J., Lin, C.-H., & Lin, L.-H. (2001). Noise and related events in a neonatal intensive care unit. *Acta Pediatr Taiwan, 42*(4), 212.

Chaudhury, H., Mahmood, A., & Valente, M. (2003). *The use of single patient rooms vs. multiple occupancy rooms in acute care environments: A review and analysis of the literature* (Unpublished report). Vancouver: Simon Fraser University.

Chhokar, R., Engst, C., Miller, A., Robinson, D., Tate, R. B., & Yassi, A. (2005). The three-year economic benefits of a ceiling lift intervention aimed to reduce health care worker injuries. *Applied Ergonomics, 36*(2), 223-229.

Clancy, C. M. (2008). Designing for safety: Evidence-based design and hospitals. *American Journal of Medical Quality, 23*(1), 66-69.

Clatworthy, S. (1981). Therapeutic play: Effects on hospitalized children. *Child Health Care, 9*(4), 108-113.

Cohen, B., Saiman, L., Cimiotti, J., & Larson, E. (2003). Factors associated with hand hygiene practices in two neonatal intensive care units. *Pediatric Infectious Diseases Journal, 22*(6), 494-499.

Cooper Marcus, C. & Barnes, M. (1999). *Healing gardens: Therapeutic benefits and design recommendations.* New York: John Wiley & Sons.

Cote, C. J., Karl, H. W., Notterman, D. A., Weinberg, J. A., & McCloskey, C. (2000). Adverse sedation events in pediatrics: Analysis of medications used for sedation. *Pediatrics, 106*(4), 633-644.

Couper, R. T., Hendy, K., Lloyd, N., Gray, N., Williams, S., & Bates, D. J. (1994). Traffic and noise in children's wards. *Medical Journal of Australia, 160*(6), 338-341.

Craddock, T. M. (2003). *The play behaviors of hospitalized children.* University of West Virginia, Morgantown.

Crowley, S., Lee, C., Tseng, C., Fogg, L. F., & Eastman, C. I. (2003). Combinations of bright light, scheduled dark, sunglasses, and melatonin to facilitate circadian entrainment to night shift work. *Journal of Biological Rhythms, 18*(6), 513-523.

Cureton-Lane, R. A. & Fontaine, D. K. (1997). Sleep in the pediatric ICU: An empirical investigation. *American Journal of Critical Care, 6*(1), 56-63.

Davidson, J. E., Powers, K., Hedayat, K. M., Tieszen, M., Kon, A. A., Shepard, E., et al. (2007). Clinical practice guidelines for support of the family in the patient-centered intensive care unit: American College of Critical Care Medicine Task Force 2004-2005. *Critical Care Medicine, 35*(2), 605-622.

DeLoach Walworth, D. (2005). Procedural-support music therapy in the healthcare setting: A cost-effectiveness analysis. *Journal of Pediatric Nursing, 20*(4).

Dill, K. & Gance-Cleveland, B. (2005). Family-centered care. *Journal for Specialists in Pediatric Nursing, 10*(4), 204-207.

Dill, K. (2006). A case for family presence. *Journal of Pediatric Nursing, 21*(2), 128-128.

Dolan, S. A., Eberhart, T., & James, J. F. (2006). Bubbles to wubbles: An investigation involving the contamination of soap bubble products at a pediatric hospital. *Journal for Specialists In Pediatric Nursing: JSPN, 11*(3), 189-195.

Donald, I. P., Pitt, K., Armstrong, E., & Shuttleworth, H. (2000). Preventing falls on an elderly care rehabilitation ward. *Clinical Rehabilitation, 14*(2), 178-185.

Drahota, A., Gal, D., & Windsor, J. (2007). Flooring as an intervention to reduce injuries from falls in healthcare settings. *Quality in Ageing, 8*(1), 3-9.

Dubbs, D. (2006). New vistas in kids' care. Family amenities and greater efficiencies emphasized in recent pediatric hospital projects. *Health Facilities Management, 19*(10), 31-34.

Eckle, N., & MacLean, S. (2001). Assessment of family-centered care policies and practices for pediatric patients in nine US emergency departments. *Journal of Emergency Nursing, 27*(3), 238-245.

Eisert, D., Kulka, L., & Moore, K. (1988). Facilitating play in hospitalized handicapped children: The design of a therapeutic play environment. *Child Health Care, 16*(3), 201-208.

Facility Guidelines Institute, AIA Academy of Architecture for Health, & U.S. Department of Health and Human Services. (2006). *Guidelines for design and construction of health care facilities.* Washington, DC: American Institute of Architects/Facility Guidelines Institute. Paper presented at Interact 2001. Japan.

Fels, D. I., Waalen, J. K., Zhai, S., & Weiss, P. L. (2001). Telepresence under exceptional circumstances: Enriching the connection to school for sick children.

Fischer, J. E., Calame, A., Dettling, A. C., Zeier, H., & Fanconi, S. (2000). Experience and endocrine stress responses in neonatal and pediatric critical care nurses and physicians. *Critical Care Medicine, 28*(9), 3281-3288.

Flynn, E. A., Barker, K. N., Gibson, J. T., Pearson, R. E., Berger, B. A., & Smith, L. A. (1999). Impact of interruptions and distractions on dispensing errors in an ambulatory care pharmacy. *American Journal of Health Systems Pharmacy, 56*(13), 1319-1325.

Flynn, E. A., Barker, K. N., Gibson, J. T., Pearson, R. E., Smith, L. A., & Berger, B. A. (1996). Relationships between ambient sounds and the accuracy of pharmacists' prescription-filling performance. *Human Factors, 38*(4), 614-622.

FMI. (2007). *FMI's construction outlook - Fourth quarter.* Raleigh, NC: FMI.

Forsythe, P. (1998). New practices in transitional care center improve outcomes for babies and their families. *Journal of Perinatology, 18*(6 pt 2 supplement), 13-17.

Fowler, E., MacRae, S., Stern, A., Harrison, T., Gerteis, M., Walker, J., et al. (1999). The built environment as a component of quality care: Understanding and including the patient's perspective. *Joint Commission Journal on Quality Improvement, 25*(7), 352-362.

Franck, L. & Callery, P. (2004). Re-thinking family-centered care across the continuum of children's healthcare. *Child: Care, Health and Development, 30*(3), 265-277.

Fudge, C. (2006, June 1). Sustainable Flooring: Renovating a Children's Hospital with Rubber. Retrieved January 10, 2008, from http://www.edcmag.com/CDA/Archives/cd710e983b8fb010VgnVCM100000f932a8c0

Gariepy, N. & Howe, N. (2003). The therapeutic power of play: Examining the play of young children with leukemia. *Child: Care, Health and Development, 29*(6), 523-537.

Gerbrands, A., Albayrak, A., & Kazemier, G. (2004). Ergonomic evaluation of the work area of the scrub nurse. *Minimally Invasive Therapy & Allied Technology, 13*(3), 142-146.

Gershon, J., Zimand, E., Lemos, R., Rothbaum, B. O., & Hodges, L. (2003). Use of virtual reality as a distractor for painful procedures in a patient with pediatric cancer: a case study. *Cyberpsychology & Behavior, 6*(6), 657-661.

Giacoia, G. P., Rutledge, D., & West, K. (1985). Factors affecting visitation of sick newborns. *Clinical Pediatrics, 24*(5), 259-262.

Giunta, F. & Rath, J. (1969). Effect of environmental illumination in prevention of hyperbilirubinemia of prematurity. *Pediatrics, 44*(2), 162-167.

Glod, C. A., Teicher, M. H., Butler, M., Savino, M., Harper, D., Magnus, E., et al. (1994). Modifying quiet room design enhances calming of children and adolescents. *Journal of the American Academy of Child and Adolescent Psychiatry, 33*(4), 558-566.

Gold, K. J., Gorenflo, D. W., Schwenk, T. L., & Bratton, S. L. (2006). Physician experience with family presence during cardiopulmonary resuscitation in children. *Pediatric Critical Care Medicine: A Journal of The Society of Critical Care Medicine and The World Federation of Pediatric Intensive and Critical Care Societies, 7*(5), 428-433.

Goldschmidt, K. A. & Gordin, P. (2006). A model of nursing care microsystems for a large neonatal intensive care unit. *Advances in Neonatal Care.*

Gosfield, A. G. & Reinertsen, J. L. (2005). The 100,000 lives campaign: Crystallizing standards of care for hospitals. *Health Affairs, 24*(6), 1560-1570.

Graven, S. N. (2004). Early neurosensory visual development of the fetus and newborn. *Clinics in Perinatology, 31*(2), 199-216.

Gray, L. & Philbin, M. (2005). Effects of the neonatal intensive care unit on auditory attention and distraction. *Clinical Perinatol, 31,* 243-260.

Greenberg, S. B., Faeber, E. N., Aspinall, C. L., & Adams, R. C. (1993). High-dose chloral hydrate sedation for children undergoing MR imaging: Safety and efficacy in relation to age. *American Journal of Roentegen Society, 161,* 639-641.

Griffin, T. (2003). Facing challenges to family-centered care. I: Conflicts over visitation. *Pediatric Nursing, 29*(2), 135-137.

Guenther, R., & Vittori, G. (2008). *Sustainable healthcare architecture.* New York: Wiley and Sons.

Gusella, J. L., Ward, A.-M., & Butler, G. S. (1998). The experience of hospitalized adolescents: How well do we meet their developmental needs. *Children's Health Care, 27*(2), 131-145.

Haiat, H., Bar-Mor, G., & Shochat, M. (2003). The world of the child: A world of play even in the hospital. *Journal of Pediatric Nursing, 18*(3), 209-214.

Hamilton, D. K., Orr, R. D., & Raboin, W. E. (2008, forthcoming). Organizational transformation: A model for joint optimization of culture change and evidence-based design. *Health Environments Research and Design Journal, 1*(3).

Harris, D. D., Shepley, M. M., White, R. D., Kolberg, K. J. S., & Harrell, J. W. (2006). The impact of single family room design on patients and caregivers: Executive summary. *Journal of Perinatology, 26,* S38-S48.

Harris, P. B., McBride, G., Ross, C., & Curtis, L. (2002). A place to heal: Environmental sources of satisfaction among hospital patients. *Journal of Applied Social Psychology, 32*(6), 1276-1299.

Healey, F. (1994). Does flooring type affect risk of injury in older in-patients? *Nursing Times, 90*(27), 40-41.

Hendrich, A. & Lee, N. (2005). Intra-unit patient transports: Time, motion, and cost impact on hospital efficiency. *Nursing Economic$, 23*(4), 157-164.

Hendrich, A. (2003). *Case Study: The impact of acuity adaptable rooms on future designs, bottlenecks and hospital capacity.* Paper presented at the Impact Conference on optimizing the physical space for improved outcomes, satisfaction and the bottom line, Atlanta.

Hendrich, A., Bender, P. S., & Nyhuis, A. (2003). Validation of the Hendrichs II falls risk model: A large concurrent case/control study of hospitalized patients. *Applied Nursing Research, 16*(1), 9-21.

Hendrich, A., Fay, J., & Sorrells, A. (2004). Effects of acuity-adaptable rooms on flow of patients and delivery of care. *American Journal of Critical Care, 13*(1), 35-45.

Henriksen, K., Isaacson, S., Sadler, B. L., & Zimring, C. M. (2007). The role of the physical environment in crossing the quality chasm. *The Joint Commission Journal on Quality and Patient Safety, 33*(11 Supplement), 68-80.

Henriksen, K., Isaacson, S., Sadler, B., & Zimring, C. (2007). The role of the physical environment in crossing the quality chasm. *The Joint Commission Journal on Quality and Patient Safety, 33*(11), 68-80.

Hignett, S. & Masud, T. (2006). A review of environmental hazards associated with in-patient falls. *Ergonomics, 5-6,* 605-616.

Hofer, C., Abreu, T., Silva, E., Sepulveda, C., Gibara, F., Lopes, N., et al. (2007). Quality of hand hygiene in a pediatric hospital in Rio de Janerio, Brazil. *Infect Control Hosp Epidemiol, 28*(5), 622-624.

Hoffman, H. G., Doctor, J. N., Patterson, D. R., Carrougher, G. J., & Furness, T. A., 3rd. (2000). Virtual reality as an adjunctive pain control during burn wound care in adolescent patients. *Pain, 85*(1-2), 305-309.

Holden, G., Bearison, D. J., Rode, D. C., Fishman, M., & Rosenberg, G. (2001). The impact of a computer network on pediatric pain and anxiety: A randomized controlled clinical trial. *Social Work in Health Care: The Journal of Health Care Social Work, 36*(2), 21-33.

Holden, G., Bearison, D. J., Rode, D. C., Rosenberg, G., & Fishman, M. (1999). Evaluating the effects of a virtual environment (Starlight Starbright programs) with hospitalized children. *Research on Social Work, 9*(3), 365-382.

Horowitz, T., Cade, B., Wolfe, J., & Czeisler, C. (2001). Efficacy of bright light and sleep/darkness scheduling in alleviating circadian maladaptation to night work. *American Journal of Physiology - Endocrinology and Metabolism, 281,* 384-391.

Humphreys, H., Johnson, E. M., Warnock, D. W., Willatts, S. M., Winter, R. J., & Speller, D. C. (1991). An outbreak of aspergillosis in a general ITU. *The Journal of Hospital Infection, 18*(3), 167-177.

Hutton, A. (2002). The private adolescent: Privacy needs of adolescents in hospitals. *Journal of Pediatric Nursing, 17*(1), 67-72.

Hutton, A. (2003). Activities in the adolescent ward environment. *Contemporary Nurse, 14,* 312-319.

Hutton, A. (2005). Issues in clinical nursing: Consumer perspectives in adolescent ward design. *Journal of Clinical Nursing, 14*(5), 537-545.

Institute for Healthcare Improvement. (2007, July 10). Transforming care at the bedside framework. Retrieved January 6, 2008, from http://www.ihi.org/NR/rdonlyres/1B99258A-D5B4-4DF5-BFD8-D334DF2E50F9/5809/VisioTCABframework0907.pdf.

Institute for Healthcare Improvement. (2008). Reaping the harvest: A review of the 5 Million Lives Campaign's first year...and a preview of what's to come. Retrieved January 5, 2008, from http://www.ihi.org/NR/rdonlyres/A528208C-8B71-4559-BFF3-F1FBDC4CD11C/0/ReapingtheHarvestBrochureFINALwebedition.pdf.

Institute of Medicine. (2000). *To err is human: Building a safer health system.* Washington, DC: National Academy Press.

Institute of Medicine. (2001). *Crossing the quality chasm: A new health system for the 21st century.* Washington, DC: National Academy Press.

Ispa, J., Barrett, B., & Yanghee, K. (1988). Effects of supervised play in hospital waiting room. *Chile Health Care, 16*(3), 195-200.

Iwata, N., Ichii, S., & Egashira, K. (1997). Effects of bright artificial light on subjective mood of shift work nurses. *Industrial Health, 35,* 41-47.

Johnson, A. N. (2001). Neonatal response to control of noise inside the incubator. *Pediatric Nursing, 27*(6), 600-605.

Jones, C. B. (2005). The costs of nurse turnover, part 2 - Application of the nursing turnover cost calculation methodology. *Journal of Nursing Administration, 35*(1), 41-49.

Jones, H. (2007, November 28). 2008 Industry forecast: Keeping pace in '08. *Construction Today.*

Joseph, A. & Ulrich, R. S. (2007). *Sound Control for Improved Outcomes in Healthcare Settings.* Concord, CA: The Center for Health Design.

Joseph, A. (2006). *The Impact of Light on Outcomes in Healthcare Settings.* Concord, CA: The Center for Health Design.

Joseph, A. (2006). *The Impact of the Environment on Infections in Healthcare Facilities.* Concord, CA: The Center for Health Design.

Joseph, A. (2007). *The role of the physical and social environment in promoting health, safety and effectiveness in the healthcare workplace.* Concord, CA: The Center for Health Design.

Joseph, A., & Fritz, L. (2006, March). Ceiling lifts reduce patient-handling injuries. *Healthcare Design, 6,* 10-13.

Judkins, S. (2003). Paediatric emergency department design: Does it affect staff, patient and community satisfaction? *Emergency Medicine (Fremantle), 15*(1), 63-67.

Junior, A. L. C., Coutinho, S. M. G., & Ferreira, R. S. (2006). Planned recreation in pediatric unit waiting room: Behavioral effects. *Cadernos de Psicologia e Educacao Paideia, 16*(33), 111-118.

Jusot, J.-F., Vanhems, P., Benzait, F., Berthelot, P., Patural, H., Teyssier, G., et al. (2003). Reported measures of hygiene and incidence rates for hospital acquired diarrhea in 31 French pediatric wards: Is there any relationship. *Infection Control and Hospital Epidemiology, 24,* 520-525.

Kapelaki, U., Fovakis, H., Dimitious, H., Perdikogianni, C., Stiakaki, E., & Kalmanti, M. (2003). A novel idea for an organized hospital/school program for children with malignancies: Issues in implementation. *Pediatric Hematology and Oncology, 20*(2), 79-87.

Kats, G. (2003). *The costs and financial benefits of green buildings: A report to California's sustainable building task force.*

Kemper, K. J., & Danhauer, S. C. (2005). Music as therapy. *Southern Medical Journal, 98*(3), 282-288.

Kennedy, K., Fielder, A., Hardy, R., Tung, B., Gordon, D., & Reynolds, J. (2001). Reduced lighting does not improve medical outcomes in very low birth weight infants. *Journal of Pediatrics, 139*(4), 527-531.

Kent, W. D., Tan, A. K., Clarke, M. C., & Bardell, T. (2002). Excessive noise levels in the neonatal ICU: Potential effects on auditory system development. *Journal of Otolaryngology, 31*(6).

Kieffer, M. & Vaughn, D. (1981). Homelike surroundings lessen stress of care for pediatric patients. *Hospitals, 55*(4), 107-111.

Kissoon, N. (2006). Family presence during cardiopulmonary resuscitation: Our anxiety versus their needs. *Pediatric Critical Care Medicine: A Journal of the Society of Critical Care Medicine and The World Federation of Pediatric Intensive and Critical Care Societies, 7*(5), 488-490.

Kohn, L., Corrigan, J., & Donaldson, M. (Eds.). (1999). *To err is human: Building a safer health system.* Washington, DC: National Academy Press.

Krug, S. E., Bojko, T., Dolan, M. A., Frush, K., O'Malley, P., Sapien, R., et al. (2006). Patient- and family-centered care and the role of the emergency physician providing care to a child in the emergency department. *Pediatrics, 118*(5), 2242-2244.

Kumari, D. N., Haji, T. C., Keer, V., Hawkey, P. M., Duncanson, V., & Flower, E. (1998). Ventilation grilles as a potential source of methicillin-resistant Staphylococcus aureus causing an outbreak in an orthopaedic ward at a district general hospital. *The Journal of Hospital Infection, 39*(2), 127-133.

Larson, E. (1988). A causal link between hand washing and risk of infection?: Examination of the evidence. *Infection Control, 9*(1), 28-36.

Larson, E., Albrecht, S., & O'Keefe, M. (2005). Hand hygiene behavior in a pediatric emergency department and a pediatric intensive care unit: Comparison of use of 2 dispenser systems. *American Journal of Critical Care, 14*(4), 304-311.

Lawson, K., Daum, C., & Turkewitz, G. (1977). Environmental characteristics of a neonatal intensive-care unit. *Child Development, 48,* 1633-1639.

Leather, P., Beale, D., Santos, A., Watts, J., & Lee, L. (2003). Outcomes of environmental appraisal of different hospital waiting areas. *Environment & Behavior, 35*(6), 842-869.

Leppamaki, S., Partonen, T., Piiroinen, P., Haukka, J., & Lonnqvist, J. (2003). Timed bright-light exposure and complaints related to shift work among women. *Scandinavian Journal of Environmental Health, 29*(1), 22-26.

Levine, K. A. (2006). *Some Benefits of Nearby Nature for Hospital Visitors: Restorative Walks in Nichols Arboretum.* University of Michigan, Ann Arbor.

Levy, G. D., Woolston, D. J., & Browne, J. V. (2003). Mean noise amounts in Level II vs Level III neonatal intensive care units. *Neonatal Network, 22*(2), 33-39.

Lewis, M., Bendersky, M., Koons, A., Hegyi, T., Hiatt, I. M., Ostfeld, B., et al. (1991). Visitation to a neonatal intensive care unit. *Pediatrics, 88*(4), 795-800.

Loewy, J., Hallan, C., Friedman, E., & Martinez, C. (2005). Sleep/sedation in children undergoing EEG testing: A comparison of chloral hydrate and music therapy. *Journal of PeriAnesthesia Nursing, 20*(5), 323-332.

Lundgren, S. & Segesten, K. (2001). Nurses' use of time in a medical-surgical ward with all-RN staffing. *Journal of Nursing Management, 9,* 13-20.

Lutz, B. D., Jin, J., Rinaldi, M. G., Wickes, B. L., & Huycke, M. M. (2003). Outbreak of invasive Aspergillus infection in surgical patients, associated with a contaminated air-handling system. *Clinical Infectious Diseases, 37*(6), 786-793.

Macnab, A., Thiessen, P., McLeod, E., & Hinton, D. (2000). Parent assessment of family-centered care practices in a children's hospital. *Children's Health Care, 29*(2), 113-128.

Malone, A. B. (1996). The effects of live music on the distress of pediatric patients receiving intravenous starts, venipunctures, injections and heel sticks. *Journal of Music Therapy, 33,* 19-33.

Malone, E. B., Mann-Dooks, J. R., & Strauss, J. (2007). *Evidence based design: Application in the MHS report.* Noblis, Inc. for the Health Facility Planning Agency of the United States Army, funded by the TRICARE Management Activity Portfolio Planning and Management Directorate.

Mangurten, J., Scott, S. H., Guzzetta, C. E., Clark, A. P., Vinson, L., Sperry, J., et al. (2006). Effects of family presence during resuscitation and invasive procedures in a pediatric emergency department. *Journal Of Emergency Nursing: JEN: Official Publication of The Emergency Department Nurses Association, 32*(3), 225-233.

Mann, N., Haddow, R., Stokes, L., Goodley, S., & Rutter, N. (1986). Effect of night and day on preterm infants in a newborn nursery. *British Medical Journal, 293*(6557), 1265-1267.

Matincheck, T. (2006). Nurses' beliefs and practices of family presence during cardiopulmonary resuscitation and invasive procedures: review of literature. *Topics in Emergency Medicine, 28*(2), 144-148.

Matthiessen, L. F., & Morris, P. (2007). *Cost of green revisited: Reexamining the feasibility and cost impact of sustainable design in the light of increased market adoption:* Davis Langdon.

McCarthy, D. & Blumenthal, D. (2006). *Committed to safety: Ten case studies on reducing harm to patients* (No. 923). New York: Commonwealth Fund.

McColl, S. L. & Veitch, J. A. (2001). Full-spectrum lighting: A review of its effects on physiology and health. *Psychological Medicine, 31,* 949-964.

McDonald, K. (2006, May). *Art while you wait.* Paper presented at the annual meeting of the Society for the Arts in Healthcare, Chicago.

McDonald, L. C., Walker, M., Carson, L., Arduino, M., Aguero, S. M., Gomez, P., et al. (1998). Outbreak of Acinetobacter spp. bloodstream infections in a nursery associated with contaminated aerosols and air conditioners. *The Pediatric Infectious Disease Journal, 17*(8), 716-722.

Megel, M. E., Houser, C. W., & Gleaves, L. S. (1998). Children's response to immunizations: Lullabies as a distraction. *Issues in Comprehensive Pediatric Nursing, 21,* 129-145.

Meyer, E. C., Coll, C. T., Lester, B. M., Boukydis, C., McDonough, S., & Oh, W. (1994). Family based intervention improves maternal psychological well-being and feeding interaction of preterm infants. *Pediatrics, 93,* 241-246.

Miller, A., Engst, C., Tate, R. B., & Yassi, A. (2006). Evaluation of the effectiveness of portable ceiling lifts in a new long-term care facility. *Applied Ergonomics, 37*(3), 377-385.

Miller, C. L., White, R., Whitman, T. L., O'Callaghan, M. F., & Maxwell, S. E. (1995). The effects of cycled versus noncycled lighting on growth and development in preterm infants. *Infant Behavior and Development, 18*(1), 87-95.

Miller, N. O., Friedman, S. B., & Coupey, S. M. (1998). Adolescent preferences for rooming during hospitalization. *Journal of Adolescent Health, 23,* 89-93.

Moore, K. A. C., Coker, K., DuBuisson, A. B., Sweet, B., & Edwards, W. H. (2003). Implementing potentially better practices for improving family-centered care in neonatal intensive care units: Successes and challenges. *Pediatrics, 111*(4), e450-e460.

Morrison, W. E., Haas, E., Shaffner, D., Garrett, E., & Fackler, J. (2003). Noise, stress, and annoyance in a pediatric intensive care unit. *Critical Care Medicine, 31*(1), 113-119.

Morrissey, J. (2004). Debugging hospitals. Technology helps track hospital-acquired infections, along with the often unreimbursed costs of treating them. *Modern Healthcare, 34*(17), 30-32.

Mulhall, A., Kelly, D., & Pearce, S. (2004). A qualitative evaluation of an adolescent cancer unit. *European Journal of Cancer Care, 13,* 16-22.

Murphy, D. & Whiting, J. (2007). *Dispelling the myths: The true cost of healthcare-associated infections.* Washington, DC: Association for Professionals in Infection Control and Epidemiology (APIC).

Naka, A., Senda, M., Tsuji, Y., & Yata, T. (2002). Architectural planning of children's hospital wards from a point of view of play environment as assessed by children. *Journal of Architecture, Planning, and Environmental Engineering,* (561), 113-120.

National Quality Forum. Serious reportable events in healthcare: 2005-2006 update. Retrieved January 6, 2008, from http://www.qualityforum.org/projects/completed/sre.

Nibert, L. & Ondrejka, D. (2005). Family presence during pediatric resuscitation: an integrative review for evidence-based practice. *Journal of Pediatric Nursing, 20*(2), 145-147.

Nolan, T. & Bisognano, M. (2006). Finding the balance between quality and cost. *Healthcare Financial Management Magazine, 60* 67-72.

O'Gorman, S. (2007). Infant-directed singing in neonatal and paediatric intensive care. *Australia and New Zealand Journal of Family Therapy, 28*(2), 100-108.

Olds, A. & Daniel, P. (1987). *Child Health Care Facilities: Design Guidelines - Literature Outline.* Bethesda, MD.

Opal, S. M., Asp, A. A., Cannady, P. B., Jr, Morse, P. L., Burton, L. J., & Hammer, P. G., 2nd. (1986). Efficacy of infection control measures during a nosocomial outbreak of disseminated aspergillosis associated with hospital construction. *Journal of Infectious Diseases, 153*(3), 634-637.

Oren, I., Haddad, N., Finkelstein, R., & Rowe, J. M. (2001). Invasive pulmonary aspergillosis in neutropenic patients during hospital construction: Before and after chemoprophylaxis and institution of HEPA filters. *American Journal of Hematology, 66*(4), 257-262.

Parsons, R. & Hartig, T. (2000). Environmental psychophysiology. In J. T. Cacioppo & L. G. Tassinary (Eds.), *Handbook of psychophysiology (2nd ed.)* (pp. 815-846). New York: Cambridge University Press.

Pass, M. & Bolig, R. (1993). A comparison of play behaviors in two child life program variations. *Child Health Care, 22*(1), 5-17.

Pati, D. & Barach, P. (in review). Impact of view on nurse well-being: An exploratory study on chronic stress, acute stress and alertness.

Pelander, T. & Leino-Kilpi, H. (2004). Quality in pediatric nursing care: Children's expectations. *Issues Compr Pediatr Nurs, 27*(3), 139-151.

Pennsylvania Health Care Cost Containment Council. (2006). *Hospital-acquired infections in Pennsylvania* (No. Issue No. 9). Harrisburg, PA: Pennsylvania Health Care Cost Containment Council.

Perkins, A. M. & Buchhalter, J. R. (2006). Optimizing patient care in the pediatric epilepsy monitoring unit. *Journal of Neuroscience Nursing, 38*(6), 416.

Peter D. Hart Research Associates. (2001). *The nurse shortage: Perspectives from current direct care nurses and former direct care nurses.* Federation of Nurses and Health Professionals.

Philbin, M. K., & Klaas, P. (2000). Hearing and behavioral responses to sound in full term newborns. *Journal of Perinatology, 20*(Supplement), 67-75.

Piserchia, E., Bragg, C., & Alvarez, M. (1982). Play and play areas for hospitalized children. *Children's Health Care, 10*(4), 135-138.

Polkki, T., Vehvilainen, K., & Pietla, A.-M. (2001). Nonpharmacological methods in relieving children's postoperative pain: A survey on hospital nurses in Finland. *Journal of Advanced Nursing, 34*(2), 483-492.

Potter, P., Boxerman, S., Wolf, L., Marshall, J., Grayson, D., Sledge, J., et al. (2004). Mapping the nursing process: A new approach for understanding the work of nursing. *Journal of Nursing Administration, 34*(2), 101-109.

Powers, K. S. & Rubenstein, J. S. (1999). Family presence during invasive procedures in the pediatric intensive care unit: A prospective study. *Arch Pediatr Adolesc Med, 153*(9), 955-958.

Premier Inc. (2006). Centers for Medicare & Medicaid Services (CMS)/Premier Hospital Quality Incentive Demonstration (HQID) project: Findings from year two. Charlotte, NC: Premier Inc.

PricewaterhouseCoopers LLP, University of Sheffield, & Queen Margaret University College - Edinburgh. (2004). *The role of hospital design in the recruitment, retention and performance of NHS nurses in England:* Commission for Architecture & the Built Environment.

Rassine, M., Gutman, Y., & Silner, D. (2004). Developing a computer game to prepare children for surgery. *Association of Periopeerative Registered Nurses, 80*(6), 1095-1196.

Reiling, J., Knutzen, B., Wallen, T., McCullough, S., Miller, R., & Chernos, S. (2004). Enhancing the traditional hospital design process: A focus on patient safety. *Joint Commission Journal on Quality and Safety, 30*(3), 115-124.

Revision to Hospital Inpatient Prospective Payment Systems—2007 FY Occupational Mix Adjustment to Wage Index; Implementation; Final Rule, 42 CFR Cong. Rec. 47870 - 48351 (2006).

Reynolds, J. D., Hardy, R. J., Kennedy, K. A., & Spencer, R. (1998). Lack of efficacy of light reduction in preventing retinopathy of prematurity. *The New England Journal of Medicine, 338*(22), 1572.

Rice, B. & Nelson, C. (2005). Safety in the pediatric ICU: The key to quality outcomes. *Critical Care Nursing Clinics of North America, 17,* 431-440.

Robb, S. L. (2000). The effect of therapeutic music interventions on the behavior of hospitalized children in isolation: Developing a contextual support model of music therapy. *Journal of Music Therapy, 37*(2), 118-146.

Rode, D. C., Capitulo, K. L., Fishman, M., & Holden, G. (1998). The therapeutic use of technology. *The American Journal of Nursing, 98*(12), 32-35.

Rollins, J. A. (2004). Evidence-based hospital design improves health care outcomes for patients, families, and staff. *Pediatric Nursing, 30*(4), 338-339.

Sacchetti, A., Paston, C., & Carraccio, C. (2005). Family members do not disrupt care when present during invasive procedures. *Academic Emergency Medicine, 12*(5), 477-479.

Sadler, B. (2006). To the class of 2005: Will you be ready for the quality revolution? *Joint Commission Journal on Quality and Patient Safety, 32*(1), 51-55.

Sadler, B. (2006a, October). The business case for building better hospitals. *Trustee Magazine.*

Said, I. & Abu Bakar, M. S. (2004). Restorative environment: Caregiver's evaluation on hospitalized children's preference towards garden versus ward in Malaysian hospitals. Paper presented at the International Symposium for Environment-Behavior Studies.

Said, I. (2003). *Garden as an environmental intervention in healing process of hospitalized children.* Paper presented at the KUSTEM Annual Seminar on Sustainability Science and Management.

Said, I., Salleh, S. S., Abu Bakar, M. S., & Mohamad, I. (2005). Caregivers' evaluation on hospitalized children's preferences concerning garden and ward. *Journal of Asian Architecture and Building Engineering, 4*(2), 331-338.

Saunders, A. N. (1995). Incubator noise: a method to decrease decibels. *Pediatric Nursing, 21*(3), 265-268.

Schneider, S. M. & Workman, M. L. (1999). Effects of virtual reality on symptom distress in children receiving chemotherapy. *CyberPsychology & Behavior, 2*(2), 125-134.

Schoenbeck, K. (2006). Transition to the private room NICU. *Neonatal Intensive Care, 19*(6), 26-28.

Seiberth, V., Linderkamp, O., Knorz, M. C., & Liesenhoff, H. (1994). A controlled clinical trial of light and retinopathy of prematurity. *American Journal of Ophthalmology, 118*(4), 492-495.

Sharkey, M. (2007a, October). Aesthetic audio systems: Designed sound environments. Health Executive Retrieved January 18, 2008, from http://www.healthexecutive.com/content/view/1502/.

Shepley, M. M. & Davies, K. (2003). Nursing unit configuration and its relationship to noise and nurse walking behavior: An AIDS/HIV unit case study. *AIA Academy Journal* Retrieved 5/26/2004 from http://www.aia.org/aah/journal/0401/article4.asp.

Shepley, M. M. (2002). Predesign and post-occupancy analysis of staff behavior in a neonatal intensive care unit. *Children's Health Care, 31*(3), 237-253.

Shepley, M. M. (2006). The role of positive distraction in neonatal intensive care unit settings. *Journal of Perinatology, 26,* S34-S37.

Shepley, M. M., Fournier, M.-A., & McDougal, K. W. (1998). *Healthcare environments for children and their families.* Dubuque, Iowa: Kendall/Hunt Publishing Company.

Sherman, S. A., Varni, J. W., Ulrich, R. S., & Malcarne, V. L. (2005). Post-occupancy evaluation of healing gardens in a pediatric cancer center. *Landscape and Urban Planning, 73*(2-3), 167-183.

Simpson, A. H. R. W., Lamb, S., Roberts, P. J., Gardner, T. N., & Evans, J. G. (2004). Does the type of flooring affect the risk of hip fracture? *Age and Ageing, 33*(3), 242-246.

Slevin, Farrington, Duffy, Daly, & Murphy, J. (2000). Altering the NICU and measuring infants' responses. *Acta Pediatr 89,* 577-581.

Smith, A., Hefley, G., & Anand, K. (2007). Parent bed spaces in the PICU: Effect on parental stress. *Pediatric Nursing.*

Smith-Coggins, R., Rosekind, M., Buccino, K., Dinges, D., & Moser, R. (1997). Rotating shiftwork schedules: Can we enhance physician adaptation to night shifts? *Academic Emergency Medicine, 4,* 951-961.

Sturdavant, M. (1960). Intensive nursing service in circular and rectangular units. *Hospitals, JAHA, 34,* 46-48, 71-78.

The Institute for Family Centered Care. (2007). Definition of patient and family centered care. Retrieved 11/20/07, 2007.

Thear, G. & Wittmann-Price, R. A. (2006). Project noise buster in the NICU: How one facility lowered noise levels when caring for preterm infants. *American Journal of Nursing, 106*(5), 64AA.

Topf, M. & Dillon, E. (1988). Noise-induced stress as a predictor of burnout in critical care nurses. *Heart Lung, 17*(5), 567-574.

Topf, M. (1989). Sensitivity to noise, personality hardiness, and noise-induced stress in critical care nurses. *Environment and Behavior, v21 n p*(6), 717-733.

Trick, W. E., Vernon, M. O., Welbel, S. F., DeMarais, P., Hayden, M. K., & Weinstein, R. A. (2007). Multicenter intervention program to increase adherence to hand hygiene recommendations and glove use and to reduce the incidence of antimicrobial resistance. *Infection Control and Hospital Epidemiology, 28*(1), 42-49.

Trites, D. K., Galbraith, F. D., Sturdavant, M., & Leckwart, J. F. (1970). Influence of nursing-unit design on activities and subjective feelings of nursing personnel. *Environment and Behavior, 2*(3), 303-334.

Tucker, A. & Spear, S. (2006). Operational failures and interruptions in hospital nursing. *Health Services Research, 41*(3), 643-662.

Uhlig, P. (2002). Reconfiguring clinical teamwork for safety and effectiveness [electronic version]. *Focus on Patient Safety, 5,* 1-2. Retrieved 9/10/06 from www.npsf.org.

Uhlig, P., Brown, J., Nason, A., Camelio, A., & Kendall, E. (2002). System innovation: Concord Hospital. *The Joint Commission Journal on Quality Improvement, 28*(12), 666-672.

Ulrich, R. & Zhu, X. (2007). Medical complications of intra-hospital patient transports: Implications for architectural design and research. *Health Environments Research & Design Journal, 1*(1), 31-43.

Ulrich, R. S. & Gilpin, L. (2003). Healing arts: Nutrition for the soul. In S. B. Frampton, L. Gilpin & P. Charmel (eds.), *Putting Patients First: Designing and Practicing Patient-centered Care* (pp. 117-146). San Francisco: Jossey-Bass.

Ulrich, R. S., Zimring, C., Joseph, A., Quan, X., & Choudhary, R. (2004). *The role of the physical environment in the hospital of the 21st century: A once-in-a-lifetime opportunity.* Concord, CA: The Center for Health Design.

Ulrich, Zimring, Zhu, DuBose, Seo, Choi, et al. (In Press). A Review of the Research Literature on Evidence-Based Healthcare Design. *Health Environments Research and Design Journal.*

Urazoe, A., Senda, M., Tsuji, Y., & Yata, T. (2001). Architectural planning of playrooms in children's hospital wards from a play-environment point of view. *Journal of Architecture, Planning, and Environmental Engineering* (550), 143-150.

Varni, J. W., Burwinkle, T. M., Dickinson, P., Sherman, S. A., Dixon, P., Ervice, J. A., et al. (2004). Evaluation of the build environment at a children's convalescent hospital: Development of the Pediatric Quality of Life Inventory parent and staff satisfaction measure for pediatric health care facilities. *Journal of Developmental and Behavioral Pediatrics, 25*(1), 10-20.

Vavili, F. (2000). Children in hospital: A design question. *World Hospital Health Services, 36*(2), 31-39.

Vessey, J. & Mahon, M. (1990). Therapeutic play and the hospitalized child. *Journal of Pediatric Nursing, 5*(5), 328-333.

Vessey, J. A., Carlson, K. L., & McGill, J. (1994). Use of distraction with children during an acute pain experience. *Nursing Research, 43*(6), 369-372.

Walch, J. M., Rabin, B. S., Day, R., Williams, J. N., Choi, K., & Kang, J. D. (2005). The effect of sunlight on post-operative analgesic medication usage: A prospective study of spinal surgery patients. *Psychosomatic Medicine, 67*(1), 156-163.

Walsh, Reitenbach, Hudson, & DePompei. (2001). Reducing light and sound in the neonatal intensive care unit: An evaluation of patient safety, staff satisfaction and costs. *Journal of Perinatology, 21,* 230-235.

Walsh, W. F., McCullough, K. L., & White, R. D. (2006). Room for improvement: Nurses' perceptions of providing care in a single room newborn intensive care setting. *Advances in Neonatal Care, 6*(5), 261-270.

Walworth, D. D. (2005). Procedural-support music therapy in the healthcare setting: A cost-effectiveness analysis. *Journal of Pediatric Nursing, 20*(4), 276-284.

Warda, L. (2005). Development and validation of a safety audit for pediatric health care facilities: First steps toward making the hospital a safer place for children. Unpublished Ph.D. dissertation, The University of Manitoba, Canada.

White, R. & Dunn. (2006). *Recommended standards for newborn ICU design.* Paper presented at the Sixth Census Conference on Newborn ICU Design. www.nd.edu/~nicudes/Recommended%20Standards%205.10%20pdf.pdf.

White, R. (2003). Individual rooms in the NICU -- an evolving concept. *Journal of Perinatology, 23*(Supplement 1), S22-S24.

Whitehouse, S., Varni, J. W., Seid, M., Cooper-Marcus, C., Ensberg, M. J., Jacobs, J. R., et al. (2001). Evaluating a children's hospital garden environment: Utilization and consumer satisfaction. *Journal of Environmental Psychology, 21*(3), 301-314.

Wishon, P. & Brown, M. (1991). Play and the young hospitalized patient. *Early Child Development and Care, 72*(1), 39-46.

Wolitzky, K., Fivush, R., Zimand, E., Hodges, L., & Rothbaum, B. O. (2005). Effectiveness of virtual reality distraction during a painful medical procedure in pediatric oncology patients. *Psychology & Health, 20*(6), 817-824.

Yassi, A., Cooper, J. E., Tate, R. B., Gerlach, S., Muir, M., Trottier, J., et al. (2001). A randomized controlled trial to prevent patient lift and transfer injuries of health care workers. *Spine, 26*(16), 1739-1746.

Ygge, B. M., Lindholm, C., & Arnetz, J. (2006). Hospital staff perceptions of parental involvement in paediatric hospital care. *Journal of Advanced Nursing, 53*(5), 534-542.

Zahr, L. K. & de Traversay, J. (1995). Premature infant responses to noise reduction by earmuffs: Effects on behavioral and physiologic measures. *Journal of Perinatology, 15*(6), 448-455.

Zimring, C. (1990). *The costs of confusion: Non-monetary and monetary costs of the Emory University Hospital wayfinding system.* Atlanta: Georgia Institute of Technology.

ADVISORY COMMITTEE

The advisory committee comprises experts from the built environment and pediatric hospital administration fields. The advisory committee's involvement included reviewing the literature review, providing written comments and participating on multiple conference calls, facilitated by Blair Sadler along with NACHRI and Center for Health Design representatives. Information from the calls and written comments were synthesized and distributed to the entire team.

The advisory committee members are:

James M. Anderson
President and Chief Executive Officer
Cincinnati Children's Hospital Medical Center

D. Kirk Hamilton, FAIA, FACHA
Associate Professor of Architecture
Center for Health Systems & Design
Texas A & M University

J. Mitchell Harris II, Ph.D.
Director of Research and Statistics
National Association of Children's Hospitals and Related Institutions

Anjali Joseph, Ph.D.
Director of Research
The Center for Health Design

Bruce Komiske
Chief of New Hospital Design and Construction
Children's Memorial Hospital

Eileen Malone
Consultant
Noblis, Inc.

Charisse S. Oland, FACHE
Consultant
Oland Consulting

Roger A. Oxendale
President and Chief Executive Officer
Children's Hospital of Pittsburgh

Annette Ridenour
President and Chief Executive Officer
Aesthetics, Inc

Ellen Schwalenstocker, Ph.D.
Director of Child Health Quality
National Association of Children's Hospitals and Related Institutions

Mardelle Shepley, AIA, ACHA
William Pena Professor
Director of the Center for Health Systems & Design
Texas A & M University

James E. Shmerling, Dr.HA.
FACHE
President and Chief Executive Officer
The Children's Hospital

Roger S. Ulrich, Ph.D.
Professorship in Health Facilities Design
Center for Health Systems & Design
Texas A & M University

Robert White, M.D.
Director, Regional Newborn Program
Memorial Hospital

About the National Association of Children's Hospitals and Related Institutions (NACHRI)

NACHRI is a nonprofit membership organization of children's hospitals with more than 218 members in the United States, Canada, Australia, China, Italy and the United Kingdom. NACHRI promotes the health and well-being of children and their families through support of children's hospitals and health systems that are committed to excellence in providing health care to children. It does so through education, research, health promotion and advocacy.

Lawrence A. McAndrews, President and CEO

Project Team:
Kristi Donovan, Associate Director, Education
J. Mitchell Harris, Ph.D., Director, Research and Statistics
Gillian Ray, Director, Public Relations
Ellen Schwalenstocker, Ph.D., Director, Child Health Quality
Cynthia Shultz Cusick, Director, Sponsorship and Corporate Relations
Sallie Strang, Director, Communications
Laurie Dewhirst Young, Assistant Director, Communications

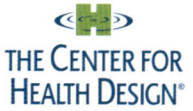

About The Center for Health Design

Founded in 1993, The Center for Health Design is a not-for-profit research and advocacy organization based in Concord, CA. Its mission is to transform health care settings into healing environments that improve outcomes through the creative use of evidence-based design. The main areas of the Center's focus are research, education, environmental standards and technical assistance. The Center is committed to sharing the evidence-based knowledge gained through its Pebble Project field-study research initiative.

Debra J. Levin, President and CEO

Project Team:
Anjali Joseph, Ph.D., Director of Research
Amy Keller, M. Arch Research Associate
Katie Kronick, Project Manager
Blair Sadler, J.D., former President and CEO, Rady Children's Hospital,
   San Diego; Senior Fellow, Institute for Healthcare Improvement
Natalie Zensius, Director of Marketing and Communications

For a copy of this publication, visit www.childrenshospitals.net